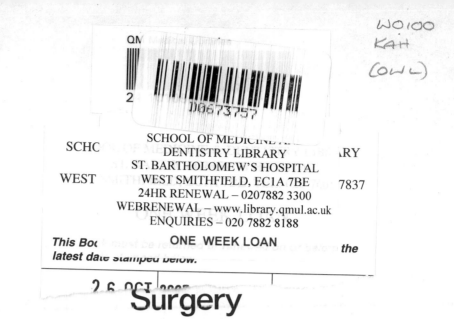
Surgery

Look for other books in this series!

In A Page Medicine

In A Page Pediatrics

In A Page Emergency Medicine

In A Page OB/GYN & Women's Health

In A Page Signs & Symptoms

In A Page Pediatric Signs & Symptoms

In A Page Surgery

Scott Kahan, MD
Intern, Franklin Square Hospital
Baltimore, MD

John J. Raves, MD
Senior Attending Staff
Division of General Surgery
Allegheny General Hospital
Pittsburgh, Pennsylvania
Assistant Professor of Surgery
Drexel University
Pittsburgh, Pennsylvania

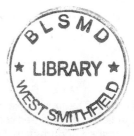

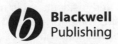
Blackwell
Publishing

© 2004 by Blackwell Publishing

Blackwell Publishing, Inc., 350 Main Street, Malden, Massachusetts 02148-5018, USA
Blackwell Publishing Ltd, 9600 Garsington Road, Oxford OX4 2DQ, UK
Blackwell Science Asia Pty Ltd, 550 Swanston Street, Carlton, Victoria 3053, Australia

03 04 05 06 5 4 3 2 1

ISBN: 1-4051-0365-5

Library of Congress Cataloging-in-Publication Data

In a page surgery / [edited by] Scott Kahan, John J. Raves.
       p. ; cm.
    Includes index.
    ISBN 1-4051-0365-5
    1. Surgery—Handbooks, manuals, etc.   2. Surgery, Operative—Handbooks, manuals, etc.
 I. Kahan, Scott.   II. Raves, John J.
    [DNLM: 1. Surgery—Handbooks.   2. Surgical Procedures, Operative—Handbooks. WO
 39 I35 2004]
    RD37.I5 2004
    617—dc21

                                                                              2003056059

A catalogue record for this title is available from the British Library

Acquisitions: Beverly Copland
Development: Kate Heinle
Production: Debra Lally
Cover design: Gary Ragaglia
Interior design: Meral Dabcovich
Typesetter: TechBooks in New Delhi, India
Printed and bound by Sheridan Books in Ann Arbor, MI

For further information on Blackwell Publishing, visit our website:
www.blackwellpublishing.com

Notice: The indications and dosages of all drugs in this book have been recommended in the
medical literature and conform to the practices of the general community. The medications
described and treatment prescriptions suggested do not necessarily have specific approval by
the Food and Drug Administration for use in the diseases and dosages for which they are recommended. The package insert for each drug should be consulted for use and dosage as
approved by the FDA. Because standards for usage change, it is advisable to keep abreast of
revised recommendations, particularly those concerning new drugs. This book is intended solely
as a review book for medical students and residents. It is not written as a guide for the intricate
clinical management of medical patients. The publisher and editor cannot accept any legal
responsibility for the content contained within this book nor any omitted information.

Table of Contents

Section 1: Gastrointestinal Disease

Colin G. Knight, MD
Mathew A. Van Deusen, MD
Nilesh A. Patel, MD

Section 2: Liver Disease

Daniel S. Salyer, MD

Table of Contents

Table of Contents

Section 7: Skin Disease
John J. Raves, MD
Brian S. Ju, MD

Section 8: Hernias
John J. Raves, MD
Brian S. Ju, MD

Section 9: Trauma
Laurel A. Omert, MD
Adrian W. Ong, MD

Section 10: Head and Neck Disease
Phillip A. Pollice, MD

Table of Contents

Table of Contents

Section 14: Neurosurgery
Jack E. Wilberger, MD, FACS

Section 15: Orthopedic Surgery
Scott Kahan, MD
Richard F. Frisch, MD

Section 16: Pediatric Surgery
Michael G. Scheidler, MD

Table of Contents

Abbreviations

A/P	Anteroposterior		DPL	Diagnostic Peritoneal Lavage
AAA	Abdominal Aortic Aneurysm		DVT	Deep Venous Thrombosis
ABG	Arterial Blood Gas		EBV	Epstein Barr Virus
ACE	Angiotensin Converting Enzyme		ECG	Electrocardiography
ACV	Assist Control Ventilation		ECMO	Extracorporeal Membrane Oxygenation
AI	Aortic Insufficiency		ED	Emergency Department
ALT	Alanine Aminotransferase		EGD	Esophagogastroduodenoscopy
APUD	Amine Precursor Uptake and Decarboxylation		EMG	Electromyography
ARDS	Adult Respiratory Distress Syndrome		ERCP	Endoscopic Retrograde Cholangiopancreatography
AS	Aortic Stenosis		ESR	Erythrocyte Sedimentation Rate
AST	Aspartate Aminotransferase		ESWL	Extracorporeal Shock Wave Lithotripsy
ATLS	Advanced Trauma Life Support		FAST	Focused Abdominal Sonographic Test
ATN	Acute Tubular Necrosis			
AV	Atrioventricular		FiO_2	Fractional Inspiration of Oxygen
AVM	Arteriovenous Malformation		FNA	Fine Needle Aspirate
AVSA	Aortic Valve Surface Area		FNH	Focal Nodular Hyperplasia
BP	Blood Pressure		FRC	Functional Residual Capacity
BPH	Benign Prostatic Hyperplasia		GCS	Glasgow Coma Scale
BUN	Blood Urea Nitrogen		GERD	Gastroesophageal Reflux Disease
Ca^+	Calcium		GFR	Glomerular Filtration Rate
CABG	Coronary Artery Bypass Grafting		GGTP	γ-Glutamyltranspeptidase
CAD	Coronary Artery Disease		GI	Gastrointestinal
CBC	Complete Blood Count		GISS	Gastrointestinal Stromal Sarcoma
CCK	Cholecystokinin		GIST	Gastrointestinal Stromal Tumor
CEA	Carcinoembryonic Antigen		GnRH	Gonadotropin Releasing Hormone
CHF	Congestive Heart Failure		GU	Genitourinary
CIS	Carcinoma In Situ		H+	Hydrogen Ion
Cl^-	Chloride Ion		HCC	Hepatocellular Carcinoma
CMV	Controlled Mandatory Ventilation		hCG	Human Chorionic Gonadotropin
CMV	Cytomegalovirus		HCT	Hematocrit
CN	Cranial Nerve		HIDA	Hepatobiliary Nuclear Scan
CNS	Central Nervous System		HIV	Human Immunodeficiency Virus
COPD	Chronic Obstructive Pulmonary Disease		hpf	High-Power Field
COX	Cyclo-Oxygenase		HTN	Hypertension
CPAP	Continuous Positive Airway Pressure		ICP	Intracranial Pressure
			ICU	Intensive Care Unit
CPK	Creatine Phosphokinase		IHISS	Hypertrophic Cardiomyopathy
CRP	C-reactive Protein		IMA	Inferior Mesenteric Artery
CSF	Cerebrospinal Fluid		INR	International Normalization Ratio
CT	Computerized Tomography		IV	Intravenous
CTA	Computerized Tomographic Angiography		IVC	Inferior Vena Cava
			IVP	Intravenous Pyelogram
CVA	Cerebrovascular Accident		LA	Left Atrium
Cx	Circumflex Coronary Artery		LAD	Left Anterior Descending Coronary Artery
CXR	Chest X-ray			
DBP	Diastolic Blood Pressure		LCIS	Lobular Carcinoma In Situ
DCIS	Ductal (intraductal) Carcinoma In Situ		LDH	Lactate Dehydrogenase
			LES	Lower Esophageal Sphincter
DIC	Disseminated Intravascular Coagulation		LFTs	Liver Function Tests
			LLQ	Left Lower Quadrant
DLT	Double Lung Transplantation		LMT	Left Main Trunk

Abbreviations

LN	Lymph Node	PTCA	Percutaneous Transluminal Coronary Angioplasty
LV	Left Ventricle		
LVA	Left Ventricular Aneurysm	PTH	Parathyroid Hormone
LVH	Left Ventricular Hypertrophy	PTT	Partial Thromboplastin Time
LWE	Local Wound Exploration	PTX	Pneumothorax
M0	No Metastases	PUD	Peptic Ulcer Disease
M1	Known Metastases	RA	Right Atrium
MAST	Military Anti-Shock Trousers	RBC	Red Blood Cell
MEN	Multiple Endocrine Neoplasia	RCA	Right Coronary Artery
MHC	Major Histocompatibility Complex	RLQ	Right Lower Quadrant
MI	Myocardial Infarction	RUQ	Right Upper Quadrant
MIBG	Metaiodobenzyl-guanidine Study (neuroectodermal tissue study)	RV	Right Ventricle
		SA	Sinoatrial
MR	Mitral Regurgitation	SAH	Subarachnoid Hemorrhage
MRA	Magnetic Resonance Angiography	SBE	Subacute Bacterial Endocarditis
MRCP	Magnetic Retrograde Cholangiopancreatography	SBP	Systolic Blood Pressure
		SCLC	Small Cell Lung Cancer
MRI	Magnetic Resonance Imaging	SIADH	Syndrome of Inappropriate Antidiuretic Hormone
MRSA	Methicillin-Resistant Staphylococcus Aureus		
		SIMV	Synchronized Intermittent Mandatory Ventilation
MS	Mitral Stenosis		
MV	Mitral Valve	SLT	Single Lung Transplantation
MVSA	Mitral Valve Surface Area	SMA	Superior Mesenteric Artery
MVA	Motor Vehicle Accident	SOB	Shortness of Breath
Mx	Unknown Metastases	SPEP	Serum Protein Electrophoresis
NG	Nasogastric	STD	Sexually Transmitted Disease
NPO	Nulla Per Os (nothing per mouth)	SVC	Superior Vena Cava
NSAID	Non-Steroidal Anti-Inflammatory Drug	TBSA	Total Body Surface Area
		TEE	Transesophageal Echocardiography
NSCLC	Non-Small Cell Lung Cancer		
NYHA	New York Heart Association	TFT	Thyroid Function Test
OPSI	Overwhelming Post-Splenectomy Infection	TIA	Transient Ischemic Attack
		TIPS	Transjugular Intrahepatic Portosystemic Shunt
OR	Operating Room		
OSA	Obstructive Sleep Apnea	TNF	Tumor Necrosis Factor
PA	Pulmonary Artery	TNM	Tumor, Node, Metastasis Staging
PCP	*Pneumocystis Carinii* Pneumonia		
PCV	Pressure-Controlled Ventilation	TSH	Thyroid Stimulating Hormone
PDA	Posterior Descending Coronary Artery	TURP	Transurethral Resection of the Prostate
PE	Pulmonary Embolus	UGI	Upper Gastrointestinal Series
PEEP	Positive End-Expiration Pressure	UPEP	Urine Protein Electrophoresis
PEG	Percutaneous Endoscopic Gastrostomy	URI	Upper Respiratory Infection
		UTI	Urinary Tract Infection
PET	Positron Emission Tomography	VACTERL	Vertebral, Anal, Cardiac, Tracheal, Esophageal, Renal, Limb
PID	Pelvic Inflammatory Disease		
PIP	Peak Inspiratory Pressure	VATS	Video-Assisted Thoracoscopy
PMN	Polymorphonuclear Cell	VRE	Vancomycin-Resistant Enterococcus
PSA	Prostate-Specific Antigen		
PSV	Pressure Support Ventilation	VSD	Ventricular Septal Defect
PT	Prothrombin Time	WBC	White Blood Cell
PTC	Percutaneous Transhepatic Cholangiogram	WHO	World Health Organization
		6-MP	6-Mercaptopurine

Contributors

Jesse D. Baer
Class of 2004
Drexel College of Medicine
Philadelphia, Pennsylvania

Rebecca Campen, MD, MS, JD
Assistant Professor of Dermatology
Harvard Medical School
Boston, Massachusetts
Attending Dermatologist
Massachusetts General Hospital
Boston, Massachusetts

Jason W. Cotter, MD
Chief Resident, General Surgery
Allegheny General Hospital
Pittsburgh, Pennsylvania

Michael L. Forbes, MD
Pediatric & Adolescent Intensivist
Assistant Professor of Pediatrics
Drexel University College of Medicine
Philadelphia, Pennsylvania
Medical Director, Inpatient Pediatric Service
Allegheny General Hospital
Pittsburgh, Pennsylvania

Richard F. Frisch, MD
Resident, Orthopedic Surgery
Albert Einstein Medical Center
Philadelphia, Pennsylvania

Christopher G. Johnnides, MD
Chief Resident, Department of Surgery
Allegheny General Hospital
Pittsburgh, Pennsylvania

Brian S. Ju, MD
Resident, General Surgery
Allegheny General Hospital
Pittsburgh, Pennsylvania

Colin G. Knight, MD
Resident, General Surgery
Allegheny General Hospital
Pittsburgh, Pennsylvania

Contributors

Jason J. Lamb, M.D.
Attending Thoracic Surgeon
Assistant Professor of Surgery
Temple University
School of Medicine
Philadelphia, Pennsylvania
Director, The Center for Lung and Thoracic Diseases
The Western Pennsylvania Hospital
Pittsburgh, Pennsylvania

John C. Lyne, MD
Attending Urologist
Department of Surgery
Allegheny General Hospital
Pittsburgh, Pennsylvania

Mary Beth Malay, MD
General Surgeon
Specializing in the Treatment of Breast Disease & Breast Cancer
Department of Human Oncology
Allegheny Cancer Center
Allegheny General Hospital
Pittsburgh, Pennsylvannia
MCP-Hahnemann School of Medicine
Philadelphia, Pennsylvania

Walter E. McGregor, MD
Fellow, Department of Cardiothoracic Surgery
Allegheny General Hospital
Pittsburgh, Pennsylvania

Ralph J. Miller, Jr., MD, FACS
Attending Urologist
Department of Surgery
Allegheny General Hospital
Pittsburgh, Pennsylvania
Assistant Professor
Department of Surgery
MCP-Hahnemann School of Medicine
Philadelphia, Pennsylvania

Laurel A. Omert, MD
Attending Surgeon
Allegheny General Hospital
Pittsburgh, Pennsylvania
Associate Professor of Surgery
Drexel University
Philadelphia, Pennsylvania

Contributors

Adrian W. Ong, MD
Attending Surgeon, Department of Surgery
Allegheny General Hospital
Pittsburgh, Pennsylvania

Nilesh A. Patel, MD
Chief Resident, General Surgery
Allegheny General Hospital
Pittsburgh, Pennsylvania

Phillip A. Pollice, MD
Senior Attending Otolaryngologist
Department of Head and Neck Surgery
Allegheny General Hospital
Pittsburgh, Pennsylvania

Daniel S. Salyer, MD
Chief Resident, General Surgery
Allegheny General Hospital
Pittsburgh, Pennsylvania

Michael G. Scheidler, MD
Surgical Fellow, Department of Pediatric Surgery
Arkansas Children's Hospital
Little Rock, Arkansas

Mathew A. Van Deusen, MD
Resident, General Surgery
Allegheny General Hospital
Pittsburgh, Pennsylvania

Jack E. Wilberger, MD, FACS
Chairman of Neurosurgery
Allegheny General Hospital
Pittsburgh, Pennsylvania
Professor of Neurosurgery
Drexel University School of Medicine
Philadelphia, Pennsylvania

Consultants

John C. Adkins, MD, FACS
Attending Surgeon
Children's Hospital of Pittsburgh
Pittsburgh, Pennsylvania
Associate Professor of Pediatric Surgery
University of Pittsburgh School of Medicine
Pittsburgh, Pennsylvania

Joseph N. Daniel, DO
Attending Orthopedic Surgeon
Albert Einstein Medical Center
Philadelphia, Pennsylvania
Director, Foot & Ankle Service
Albert Einstein Medical Center
Philadelphia, Pennsylvania

Preface

The *In A Page* series was designed to streamline the vast amount of material that saturates the study of medicine, providing students, residents, and health professionals a high yield, big picture overview of the most important clinical medical topics. *In A Page Surgery* is the fourth handbook of this series. We expect this book to be especially useful for 3rd and 4th year medical students, interns, and other health professionals.

We have tried to cover the most important surgical topics in a manner that facilitates quick retrieval and easy understanding and we have included the latest, evidenced-based information.

We have followed the general format of the previous *In A Page* handbooks. In addition, we included introduction pages that precede nearly every chapter, which give information on relevant anatomy and useful facts. Certainly, this book is not intended as a detailed anatomy text. Rather than present detailed anatomic discussions in these pages, we have picked out only what we believe to be the most useful surgical anatomic pearls. Those who require more intricate anatomic detail should consult an anatomy text.

The vast majority of surgery occurs outside the operating room—from the workup and identification of diseases to non-operative interventions and patient management. As such, rather than focusing on the details of operative procedures, we chose to concentrate on the "big picture" of each disease, which is centered on understanding the etiology and pathophysiology, forming a solid differential diagnosis, and performing an efficient workup. Since the primary objectives of students and early residents are non-surgical, we believe this approach will afford readers a better understanding of the approach to surgical disease. For example, students and interns generally do not need to know the specific steps of the Whipple procedure nor the exact gauge of needle used for a liver biopsy. Alternatively, they should understand the significance of the Whipple procedure (i.e., purpose, indications, and goals of surgery) and what criteria indicate the need for a liver biopsy.

As in the initial books of the series, we were constrained by the size of the template and the need to keep each disease within a single page. We had to be quite succinct in our explanations and descriptions and we sacrificed details in some cases, such as drug dosages.

We are certain that the final product will be a very effective resource. Reviews from medical students and residents have been very positive. We anticipate that this book will be a valuable tool in the hospital, as board review, and for independent study. We welcome any comments, questions, or suggestions. Please address correspondence to drkahan@yahoo.com.

Acknowledgments

Certainly, the greatest strength of this book is its diverse group of authors, a collection of residents, fellows, attending surgeons, and specialists. We sincerely thank everyone who worked with us.

We are also grateful to the staff at Blackwell Publishing, especially Kate Heinle, Bev Copland, and Debra Lally. Their help during the course of this project was invaluable.

Gastrointestinal Disease

Section 1

COLIN G. KNIGHT, MD
MATHEW A. VAN DEUSEN, MD
NILESH A. PATEL, MD

1. GI Anatomy, Facts, and Pearls

- The gastrointestinal tract, consisting of the esophagus, stomach, duodenum, jejunum, ileum, colon, and rectum is designed for digestion and absorption of foods in order to sustain growth and survival
- The upper GI tract includes structures proximal to the Ligament of Treitz (esophagus, stomach, and duodenum)
- The lower GI tract includes the bowel distal to the Ligament of Treitz (jejunum, ileum, colon, rectum)

Esophagus
- Mucosal lining is normally composed of squamous epithelium
- The upper one-third of the esophagus is composed of skeletal muscle; the middle one-third transitions from skeletal muscle to smooth muscle; the lower one-third is composed of smooth muscle
- There is no serosa of the esophagus
  - Tumors that penetrate through the esophageal muscle layer will directly enter the mediastinum
  - Increased incidence of anastomotic leaks secondary to the absence of the protecting seroza
- The lower esophageal sphincter is not a true sphincter, but rather a high pressure zone that protects the esophagus from gastric acid

Stomach
- The fundus and body contain acid-secreting parietal cells
- The antrum is responsible for peristalsis and "grinding" of food particles
- The antrum is the site of G cells, which produce gastrin to stimulate parietal cells to produce acid
- The pylorus is the sphincter muscle that separates the stomach from the duodenum and allows passage of food to the duodenum
- The stomach is extremely well vascularized
- The left and right vagus nerves descend along the esophagus and become the anterior and posterior vagal trunks, respectively

Duodenum
- Proximal small bowel beginning just beyond the pylorus and extending to the Ligament of Treitz
- The majority of the duodenum is retroperitoneal
- The common bile duct and the main pancreatic duct (Wirsung) enter the small bowel at the ampulla of Vater, located in the second portion of the duodenum
- The accessory pancreatic duct (Santorini) is present in 60% of the population and enters the duodenum just proximal to the ampulla of Vater

Jejunum
- The middle one-third of the small bowel, beginning at the Ligament of Treitz
- The entire jejunum is intraperitoneal
- The jejunum is the site of maximum absorption of most ingested foods

Ileum
- The distal one-third of the small bowel
- The entire ileum is intraperitoneal
- The mucosa of the ileum is less permeable than the jejunum, requiring greater use of active-transport mechanisms (i.e., there are specific absorption receptors for vitamin B_{12} and bile salts)

Colon
- Primary functions are the reabsorption of water and sodium, secretion of potassium and bicarbonate, and storage of fecal material
- The ascending and descending colon are retroperitoneal; the transverse and sigmoid colon are intraperitoneal

Hormones and Neurotransmitters of the Small Intestine
- Cholecystokinin (CCK) is responsible for contraction of the gallbladder, relaxation of the sphincter of Oddi, and stimulation of pancreatic exocrine secretion
- Secretin stimulates pancreatic secretion in response to duodenal acid
- Somatostatin regulates the release of gastric acid and gastrin, and stimulates pancreatic islet cells
- Gastric inhibitory polypeptide is released by the duodenum and jejunum and acts to augment insulin response after meals

Blood Supply of the Gastrointestinal Tract
- The celiac trunk provides arteries that supply the lower esophagus, stomach, and proximal duodenum
  - The stomach is supplied by the left and right gastric arteries, left and right gastroepiploic arteries, and the short gastric arteries
  - The pylorus is supplied by the gastroduodenal arteries
  - The proximal duodenum is supplied by the superior pancreatico-duodenal arteries
- The superior mesenteric artery supplies the duodenum, jejunum, ileum, cecum, ascending (right) colon, and proximal transverse colon
- The inferior mesenteric artery supplies the distal transverse colon, the descending (left) colon, sigmoid colon, and the upper and middle rectum
- The internal iliac artery supplies the lower rectum

2. Acute Abdomen

Etiology/Pathophysiology

- Acute onset (<10 days) of sudden, severe abdominal pain
  - Visceral pain is characterized by diffuse, colicky, crampy pain secondary to distention or contraction of a hollow abdominal organ (e.g., intestine, stomach)
  - Parietal (somatic) pain is more localized and constant than visceral pain; occurs secondary to inflammation and direct irritation of the peritoneum
- Distinguish etiologies requiring emergent or urgent surgical intervention (i.e., a *surgical* abdomen) from non-emergent causes
  - Acute surgical emergencies include ruptured aortic aneurysm, perforated viscus (e.g., diverticulitis, peptic ulcer), appendicitis, intestinal obstruction, ischemic bowel, ruptured ectopic pregnancy
  - Non-surgical conditions include renal colic, pelvic inflammatory disease (PID), pancreatitis
- Non-abdominal causes of pain that mimic an acute abdomen are numerous and may include myocardial infarction, atypical angina, pericarditis, pneumonia, pulmonary embolus, pelvic pathology (e.g., pelvic inflammatory disease, ovarian torsion)

Differential Dx

- Appendicitis
- Cholecystitis
- Diverticulitis
- Gastroenteritis
- Pancreatitis
- PID
- Biliary or renal colic
- Ruptured abdominal aortic aneurysm
- Peptic ulcer disease
- Gastritis
- Bowel obstruction
- Ischemic bowel
- Ectopic pregnancy
- Intussusception
- Pneumonia
- Myocardial infarction
- Pulmonary embolus
- Ovarian torsion

Presentation/Signs & Symptoms

- Crampy, colicky pain that occurs in waves implies distention of a hollow viscus (e.g., renal colic, intestinal obstruction)
- Constant, localized pain implies inflammation (e.g., appendicitis, diverticulitis, cholecystitis)
- Associated symptoms may include nausea, vomiting, constipation or diarrhea, anorexia, dysuria
- Hypotension and shock may be present
- In general, patients who present with extremely severe pain of immediate onset require surgical intervention
- Atypical presentations are common in elderly, infant, alcoholic, and immunocompromised patients

Diagnostic Evaluation

- History and physical exam will narrow the differential and determine whether the patient requires emergent surgery
  - Nature of pain (visceral versus parietal), location, onset, duration, intensity, similarity to past episodes, and aggravating and alleviating factors
  - Physical exam should note rebound tenderness, guarding, bowel sounds, distension, presence of a mass, blood on rectal exam, cervical or adnexal tenderness
- Initial tests should include CBC, electrolytes, liver function tests, amylase/lipase, urinalysis, and pregnancy test
- Imaging studies may be necessary to establish a diagnosis
  - Plain abdominal X-rays may reveal obstruction, perforation (free air), and other pathology
  - Ultrasound is indicated if biliary tract disease, aortic aneurysm, or ectopic pregnancy is suspected
  - Abdominal CT will often establish the diagnosis for urolithiasis, aortic aneurysm, diverticulitis, appendicitis

Treatment/Management

- Hemodynamically unstable patients require immediate resuscitation
  - Replace volume with normal saline and possibly a blood transfusion
  - Evidence of hemorrhage (e.g., ruptured AAA, ruptured ectopic pregnancy) or early sepsis (e.g., perforated diverticulitis, perforated bowel) may represent a life-threatening emergency that requires urgent surgical intervention
- Place NG tube for obstruction or persistent vomiting
- Administer broad-spectrum empiric antibiotics if suspect a perforated viscus or intra-abdominal infection
- Direct treatment towards the specific condition (see individual entries)

Prognosis/Complications

- Prompt diagnosis and appropriate treatment generally results in a good prognosis

3. Upper GI Bleeding

Etiology/Pathophysiology

- Involves a bleeding source proximal to the Ligament of Treitz (which separates the duodenum from the jejunum)
- A spectrum of upper GI bleeding can be from occult hemorrhage presenting as anemia to acute, life-threatening hemorrhage
  - Sources of life-threatening upper GI bleeding include peptic ulcer disease (most common cause of upper GI bleeding), esophageal varices, and Mallory-Weiss tears
- Esophageal etiologies include esophageal varices and esophagitis
- Gastric etiologies include gastric ulcer, gastritis, Mallory-Weiss tear, Dieulafoy's lesion (erosion of mucosa overlying an artery in the stomach causes necrosis of the arterial wall and resultant hemorrhage), arteriovenous malformations, gastric varices (secondary to splenic vein thrombosis), and benign or malignant tumors
- Duodenal etiologies include duodenal ulcers, erosion of a pancreatic tumor into the duodenum, and aortoenteric fistula (common following AAA repair; a small herald bleed often precedes massive hemorrhage)
- Systemic etiologies include leukemia, hemophilia, thrombocytopenia, coagulopathy or anticoagulation therapy, and hereditary hemorrhagic telangiectasia

Differential Dx

- Lower GI bleeding
- Nasopharyngeal or oropharyngeal sources of bleeding
- Systemic bleeding disorders (e.g., hemophilia, excessive anticoagulation, thrombocytopenia)

Presentation/Signs & Symptoms

- Symptoms range from occult, microscopic bleeding to frank bloody vomitus or bloody stools
- Hematemesis
- Coffee ground emesis
- Melena (dark, tarry stools)
- Hematochezia (bright red blood per rectum) indicates a lower GI bleed or a brisk upper GI bleed
- Hypovolemia due to hemorrhage (e.g., pallor, dizziness, weakness, tachycardia, syncope) and signs of shock (e.g., hypotension) may be present
- Non-specific complaints may include dyspnea, abdominal cramps, chest pain, and fatigue

Diagnostic Evaluation

- Nasogastric tube can be placed to verify blood in the upper GI tract
  - Lower GI bleeding can only be assumed if nasogastric aspirate is non-bloody and bilious (implies duodenal fluid has been sampled and is not bleeding)
- Upper GI endoscopy (EGD) is diagnostic and potentially therapeutic
  - Identifies the source of bleeding in 90% of patients
- If too much blood is present to identify a specific source of bleeding by endoscopy, a celiac and superior mesenteric angiogram is indicated to search for the source of bleeding
- If patient has a known aortic graft (prior aneurysm repair or aortic occlusive disease), a high index of suspicion for an aortoenteric fistula
- Coagulation workup may be indicated, including PT/PTT/INR, bleeding time, and platelet count

Treatment/Management

- Ensure adequate airway, breathing, and circulation
- Establish two large bore IVs, begin rapid IV fluid administration, type and cross match, correct coagulopathies if present, and consider blood transfusion
- Medical control of bleeding may be accomplished by IV octreotide infusion
- Emergent endoscopic control of bleeding may include injection of vasoconstrictors (e.g., epinephrine), injection of sclerosing agents, electrocautery, laser photocoagulation, or application of hemoclips
- Angiographic visualization of the bleeding vessel with subsequent embolization
- Surgical control of bleeding if all else fails; however, the surgeon must have an idea of the site of bleeding (by endoscopy or angiography) before beginning intervention

Prognosis/Complications

- All patients with systolic blood pressure <100, tachycardia, >4 units of blood transfused, or active bleeding should be admitted to an intensive care unit
- Prognosis depends on the underlying source of the bleed
- Overall mortality of 10%

4. Lower GI Bleeding

Etiology/Pathophysiology

- Lower GI bleeding occurs distal to the Ligament of Treitz (which separates the duodenum from the jejunum)
- A spectrum of lower GI bleeding can be from occult hemorrhage presenting as anemia to acute, life-threatening hemorrhage
  - Sources of life-threatening lower GI bleeding include diverticular hemorrhage, angiodysplasia (arteriovenous malformation), and aortoenteric fistula (GI bleeding in a patient with past aortic surgery should be assumed to be an aortoenteric fistula secondary to an infected aortic stent until proven otherwise—they often have a small herald bleed that precedes massive hemorrhaging)
- Small bowel etiologies include aortoenteric fistula, small bowel tumor, Meckel's diverticulum, and angiodysplasia
- Colonic etiologies include diverticular hemorrhage, angiodysplasia, colon cancer, polyps, and colitis
- Rectal etiologies include polyps, hemorrhoids, and rectal cancer

Differential Dx

- Upper GI bleeding
- Systemic bleeding disorders (e.g., hemophilia, excessive anticoagulation, thrombocytopenia)

Presentation/Signs & Symptoms

- Blood in the stool ranges from occult, microscopic bleeding to frank bloody stools
- Melena (dark, tarry stool)
- Hematochezia (bright red blood per rectum) indicates a lower GI bleed or a brisk upper GI bleed
- Hypovolemia due to hemorrhage (e.g., pallor, dizziness, weakness, tachycardia, syncope) and signs of shock (e.g., hypotension) may be present
- Nonspecific complaints may include dyspnea, abdominal cramps, chest pain, and fatigue

Diagnostic Evaluation

- Rectal examination for melena and hematochezia
- Rule out upper GI bleeding by nasogastric tube aspiration or upper GI endoscopy
- Draw blood for type and cross match, PT/PTT/INR, CBC, and chemistries
- In acute blood loss, hematocrit and hemoglobin may still be normal due to dehydration and hemoconcentration
- Colonoscopy is usually the test of choice
- Angiography may be diagnostic and therapeutic for heavy bleeding (only positive during active bleeding)
- Tagged RBC scan is very helpful for Meckel's diverticula; otherwise non-specific but may give a clue to the site of bleeding

Treatment/Management

- Ensure adequate airway, breathing, and circulation
- Establish two large bore IVs, begin rapid IV fluid administration, type and cross match, correct coagulopathies if present, and consider blood transfusion
- Definitive treatment depends on the specific cause
  - Diverticular hemorrhage may require resection
  - Angiodysplasia may be treated by endoscopy with electrocautery or surgical resection
  - Meckel's diverticula requires excision or resection
  - Aortoenteric fistula requires repair of bowel, graft excision, and extra-anatomic bypass (e.g., axillo-bifemoral graft)
  - Colon cancer requires resection
  - Colon and rectal polyps require excision or resection
  - Colitis is usually treated medically

Prognosis/Complications

- All patients with systolic blood pressure <100, tachycardia, >4 units of blood transfused, or active bleeding should be admitted to an intensive care unit
- Prognosis depends on the underlying source of the bleed
- Angiodysplasia and diverticular bleeding have high risks of repeat bleeding; elective resection should be considered
- Patients with aortoenteric fistula have >50% mortality even with appropriate surgical intervention

5. Achalasia

Etiology/Pathophysiology

- Achalasia is the most common primary esophageal motility disorder
- Due to an absence of esophageal smooth muscle peristalsis, increased lower esophageal sphincter (LES) resting pressure, and failure of the LES to relax in response to a bolus of food
- Results in functional obstruction with esophageal dilatation (esophagus is widened and abnormally lengthened)
- Uncertain etiology (possibly a neurodegenerative disorder)
- Affects 1 in 100,000 people in the U.S.
- Usually manifests between 20 and 40 years of age, but may be seen in infancy and early childhood
- Distinguish achalasia from other disorders of esophageal motility
  - Diffuse esophageal spasm: Uncoordinated, high amplitude esophageal contractions
  - Nutcracker esophagus: Exceedingly high amplitude esophageal contractions
  - Strictures: Secondary to ingestion of caustic agents or longstanding gastroesophageal reflux or esophagitis

Differential Dx

- Diffuse esophageal spasm
- Nutcracker esophagus
- Strictures
- Hypertensive lower esophageal sphincter
- Chagas' disease (*Trypanosoma cruzi* infection resulting in achalasia, megacolon, and cardiomyopathy)
- Scleroderma
- Primary muscle dysfunction (e.g., myotonic dystrophy)
- Metabolic disorders that affect muscle function (e.g., hypothyroidism)
- Esophageal cancer

Presentation/Signs & Symptoms

- Progressive dysphagia (solids and liquids) is the most common symptom
- Substernal chest pain
- Regurgitation of undigested food
- Weight loss
- Aspiration and respiratory symptoms secondary to esophageal retention, regurgitation, and overflow into trachea
- Recurrent aspiration pneumonia
- Bloating
- Inability to burp

Diagnostic Evaluation

- Chest X-ray reveals mediastinal widening with possible air-fluid level
- Barium esophagram reveals marked dilatation of the esophagus and a narrowed, tapered ("bird beak") distal esophagus
  - Longstanding achalasia may result in a lengthened, tortuous esophagus ("sigmoid esophagus")
- Manometry is the gold standard to diagnose achalasia
  - Reveals high LES resting pressure, incomplete relaxation upon swallowing, failure of peristalsis
  - Elevated resting pressure in the body of the esophagus may also be present
- Upper GI endoscopy with biopsy is required to rule out esophageal cancer, esophagitis, and strictures

Treatment/Management

- Medical therapy (calcium channel blockers, nitrates, sildenafil) may give short-term improvement of symptoms
- Pneumatic dilatation of the LES is effective in >60% of patients
- Botulinum toxin injections is of questionable efficacy and must be repeated every few months
- Surgical treatment consists of esophagomyotomy (Heller myotomy), with sectioning of the LES
  - Laparoscopy is preferred to open thoracotomy or laparotomy
  - Commonly includes an anti-reflux procedure since an effective myotomy predisposes to reflux
  - Best results are obtained by an abdominal laparoscopic myotomy with an anti-reflux procedure

Prognosis/Complications

- Pneumatic dilatation is effective in 60% of patients after one dilatation, and 80% after two dilatations
  - 2–15% risk of perforation (increased by repeated dilatations and prior botulinum toxin injection)
- Botulinum injections are falling out of favor
  - Ineffective in nearly 40% of patients
  - Required multiple injections
  - Scarring secondary to injections results in higher risk of complications following pneumatic dilatation or surgery
- Surgery has a 3–4% complication rate (pneumothorax and esophageal mucosal perforation)
- Significantly increased risk of esophageal carcinoma

6. Esophageal Varices

Etiology/Pathophysiology

- Esophageal varices develop from prolonged or severe cases of portal hypertension
  - Portosystemic venous collaterals develop to decompress the portal system
  - Collateral porto-caval bypass channels become engorged and portal blood flow is diverted through the coronary veins of the stomach into the esophageal venous plexus and eventually into the caval circulation
- Esophageal varices themselves do not cause problems—however, their potential rupture and hemorrhage pose a life-threatening complication
- Accounts for 10% of upper GI bleeds—most common causes of upper GI bleed are peptic ulcers, gastritis, and mucosal tears
- Most commonly seen in the U.S. in alcoholic cirrhosis patients; hepatic schistosomiasis, though rare in the U.S., is the most common worldwide cause of esophageal varices
- Nearly 50% of cirrhotic patients will develop esophageal varices; of these patients, nearly 50% will have variceal hemorrhage within 1–2 years

Differential Dx

- Duodenal/gastric ulcer
- Diffuse erosive gastritis
- Gastric varices
- Mallory-Weiss tear
- Gastric carcinoma
- Esophagitis
- Esophageal carcinoma
- Dieulafoy's lesion

Presentation/Signs & Symptoms

- Rupture of varices results in painless but massive hematemesis
  - "Coffee ground" emesis and melena are less likely
- Signs of volume depletion (e.g., pallor, tachycardia, hypotension)
- Physical signs associated with liver cirrhosis and portal hypertension may be present, including hepatomegaly, splenomegaly, ascites, jaundice, palmar erythema, clubbing of fingers, spider angiomata, and caput medusae

Diagnostic Evaluation

- Initial management is similar to all upper GI bleeding (see "Upper GI Bleeding" entry)
- Upper GI endoscopy (EGD) should be performed immediately after the patient is stabilized
  - Will identify varices and source of hemorrhage and rule out other potential causes of bleeding
  - Patients with cirrhosis and known varices will have a non-variceal source of bleeding in one-third of cases (most commonly peptic ulcer disease or gastritis)

Treatment/Management

- Initial resuscitation with IV fluids, blood replacement, correction of coagulopathies, and hemodynamic monitoring
- If variceal hemorrhage is identified on endoscopy, sclerotherapy or esophageal banding are done
- IV octreotide should then be administered
- In cases of persistent bleeding, balloon tamponade via a Sengstaken-Blakemore tube may be used
- If bleeding continues, consider emergent TIPS (Transjugular Intrahepatic Portosystemic Shunt) or surgical porto-caval shunting to decompress the portal system
- Liver transplantation may be indicated if significant liver dysfunction is present

Prognosis/Complications

- Variceal bleeding rarely subsides spontaneously; nearly always requires intervention
- 40% mortality with the first episode of variceal bleeding if not adequately treated
- Recurrence occurs within 1 year in >50% of survivors; similar mortality rate for each episode
- Balloon tamponade carries a risk of aspiration and esophageal perforation
  - Endotracheal intubation is usually recommended prior to insertion of balloon

7. Esophageal Cancer

Etiology/Pathophysiology

- Squamous cell carcinoma is very common worldwide (35/100,000 cases in high risk populations) but less common in the U.S. (3/100,000)
  - Associated with alcohol and tobacco use, vitamins A and C deficiency, achalasia, nitrosamines, and molds
  - Typically multifocal, locally infiltrating, and aggressive
- Adenocarcinoma is much more common in the U.S. than in other countries
  - Since the esophageal mucosa is composed of squamous cells, adenocarcinoma can only occur at the gastroesophageal junction or in cases of Barrett's metaplasia, wherein columnar epithelium has replaced the normal squamous epithelium in the distal esophagus
  - Risk of adenocarcinoma increases 40-fold in cases of Barrett's metaplasia (adenocarcinoma develops in Barrett's at 1% per year)
  - Barrett's esophagus occurs in 10% of patients with chronic reflux disease
  - Associated with transmural esophageal involvement, lymphatic spread, and aggressive behavior

Differential Dx

- Achalasia
- Diffuse esophageal spasm
- Scleroderma
- GERD
- Esophageal web or ring
- Benign stricture
- Dysphagia lusoria (obstruction secondary to the right subclavian artery passing behind the esophagus)

Presentation/Signs & Symptoms

- Insidious onset—most patients present at late stages of disease
- Progressive dysphagia for solids (90% of cases); patients tend to alter their diets from solid to liquid foods
- Weight loss, malnutrition, dehydration
- Respiratory symptoms (e.g., choking, aspiration, pneumonia) due to aspiration or direct tumor invasion of the tracheobronchial tree
- Cough, horseness, and/or hematemesis
- Pain/retrosternal discomfort
- Paraneoplastic syndromes may include hypercalcemia secondary to ectopic secretion of parathyroid hormone

Diagnostic Evaluation

- History and physical exam should evaluate for the degree of dysphagia (e.g., solids versus liquids), subjective location of swallowing difficulty (cervical esophagus versus thoracic esophagus versus distal esophagus), presence of lymphadenopathy, and the presence of abdominal masses or hepatomegaly
- Upper GI endoscopy with biopsy is diagnostic
- Barium esophagogram
- CT, bronchoscopy, and endoscopic ultrasound (most accurate) are used for staging and to evaluate for metastases and local invasion
- Additional evaluation may include a fine needle aspiration of metastatic lesions

Treatment/Management

- Treatment is primarily palliative
- Surgical resection is rarely curative but may restore patency of the esophagus
  - Total esophagectomy for squamous cell carcinoma (with reconstruction using either the stomach or colon)
  - Esophagogastrectomy for adenocarcinoma
- Esophageal dilation or stenting is indicated for patients with esophageal obstruction or tracheoesophageal fistula
- Radiation or chemotherapy may marginally improve survival and/or temporarily relieve dysphagia
- Laser and photodynamic therapy

Prognosis/Complications

- Both squamous and adenocarcinomas have an extremely poor prognosis
  - Squamous: 5-year survival <10%
  - Adenocarcinoma: 5-year survival <5%
- 75% of patients have cervical or supraclavicular nodal involvement at time of presentation

8. Hiatal Hernia

Etiology/Pathophysiology

- Herniation of the stomach through a widened esophageal hiatus of the diaphragm
- Sliding hiatal hernia (90% of cases) is an upward migration of the gastroesophageal junction through the esophageal hiatus and into the thorax, most often caused by stretching of esophageal hiatus
- Paraesophageal hiatal hernia is a "rolling" of the gastric fundus upward through the esophageal hiatus and into the thorax, with normal position of the gastroesophageal junction
    - Paraesophageal hernias have a significantly increased risk of volvulus and strangulation
- Classification system includes type I (sliding hiatal hernia), type II (paraesophageal hiatal hernia), type III (combined sliding and paraesophageal), or type IV (herniation of stomach and additional intra-abdominal organ, such as colon, spleen, or omentum)

Differential Dx

- Myocardial ischemia or infarction
- GERD
- Peptic ulcer disease
- Chemical or infectious esophagitis
- Esophageal spasm
- Achalasia
- Aortic dissection
- Costochondritis

Presentation/Signs & Symptoms

- Sliding hiatal hernias are often asymptomatic
    - Incompetence of the gastroesophageal junction may result in reflux, causing symptoms of GERD (e.g., heartburn, cough, regurgitation, dysphagia)
- Paraesophageal hernias are also often asymptomatic but may present with severe ischemic symptoms if volvulus or incarceration of the stomach occurs
    - Since the gastroesophageal junction is intact, reflux rarely occurs
    - Obstructive symptoms (e.g., dysphagia, postprandial fullness, heartburn, dyspnea) may signal impending volvulus
    - Hematemesis may occur

Diagnostic Evaluation

- Upright chest X-ray may reveal a retrocardiac shadow or widening
    - Presence of an air-fluid level behind the heart usually represents a paraesophageal hernia
    - Presence of a nasogastric tube that appears to enter the abdomen but then curves back to the chest is highly suggestive of a paraesophageal hernia
- Barium swallow or upper GI series is usually diagnostic to differentiate the type of hiatal hernia and may rule out other pathology
- Upper GI endoscopy (EGD) allows direct visualization of the hernia and evaluation of the esophageal and gastric mucosa
- Chest and abdominal CT scans are often diagnostic and provide excellent anatomic information

Treatment/Management

- Sliding hernias rarely require treatment; if symptoms of associated reflux are present, treatment is directed at correcting the reflux disease (see "Gastroesophageal Reflux Disease" entry)
- Treatment of paraesophageal hernias is always operative, regardless of severity of symptoms, due to the risk of gastric volvulus or incarceration
    - Surgical treatment includes reducing of the stomach into the abdominal cavity, repairing the esophageal hiatus, and possibly an anti-reflux procedure
    - Gastropexy (intra-abdominal fixation of the stomach) is considered if gastric emptying is abnormal

Prognosis/Complications

- Infarction, bleeding, and perforation may occur in up to 25% of patients with paraesophageal hernias
- Elective surgical repair of a paraesophageal hernia carries a low operative mortality; however, an emergency repair for infarction or perforation of the stomach carries nearly 20% operative mortality

9. Gastroesophageal Reflux Disease

Etiology/Pathophysiology

- Inflammation and irritation of the esophageal mucosa due to reflux of gastric contents
- Defective lower esophageal sphincter mechanism may be present, including inappropriate sphincter relaxation, inadequate sphincter size, or abnormal sphincter position
  - Inappropriate LES relaxation may be exacerbated by alcohol, smoking, fatty foods, caffeine, chocolate, pregnancy, medications (e.g., anticholinergics, calcium channel blockers)
  - Ineffective esophageal clearance of gastric reflux material and gastric emptying abnormalities also predispose to GERD
- GERD is the most common upper GI disorder in western nations (up to 10% of the U.S. population has daily symptoms; 15–30% have symptoms at least once per month)
- Often associated with hiatal hernia

Differential Dx

- Gastritis
- Peptic ulcer disease
- Angina
- Esophageal motility disorders (e.g., achalasia, diffuse esophageal spasm)
- Esophageal cancer
- Gastric cancer

Presentation/Signs & Symptoms

- Heartburn
- Persistent, non-productive cough (GERD is the second most common cause of chronic cough in non-smokers)
- Regurgitation
- Dysphagia
- Hoarseness due to reflux laryngitis, repetitive throat clearing, hiccups
- Full feeling in throat
- Exacerbation of asthma symptoms

Diagnostic Evaluation

- History and physical exam should rule out symptoms that suggest a potentially serious etiology (e.g., nausea, vomiting, weight loss, blood in stool, true chest pain, dysphagia, anemia, long duration of symptoms, age >50)
- In most cases, a therapeutic trial of lifestyle changes, antacids, H2 blockers, or proton pump inhibitors is indicated to diagnose GERD
- Diagnostic testing may include an upper GI series with barium swallow, endoscopy, 24-hour pH monitoring, esophageal manometry, and motility studies
  - Upper GI series will evaluate for anatomic causes and/or complications of GERD (e.g., hiatal hernia, strictures)
  - Endoscopy allows direct visualization and biopsy to document esophagitis and/or Barrett's esophagus
  - 24-hour pH monitoring will diagnose reflux by correlating esophageal pH with symptom onset
  - Esophageal manometry diagnoses an ineffective LES

Treatment/Management

- Lifestyle modifications are the initial therapy for mild disease, including weight loss, dietary changes to eliminate predisposing agents, avoidance of alcohol and tobacco, avoidance of food within 4 hours of bedtime, and sleeping with head elevated
- Anti-ulcer/antacid medications are the mainstay of medical therapy
  - H2 blockers are first line therapy in mild disease
  - Proton pump inhibitors
- Anti-reflux surgery (laparoscopic or open fundoplication) provides a definitive treatment
  - Indications for surgery include presence of GERD complications (e.g., stricture, Barrett's metaplasia, development of adenocarcinoma), if symptoms persist despite maximal medical therapy, or in patients who wish to avoid lifelong medical therapy

Prognosis/Complications

- Complications of GERD include esophageal ulcers, stricture formation, Barrett's esophagus with risk of esophageal adenocarcinoma, and pulmonary complications (e.g., laryngitis, bronchitis, recurrent aspiration pneumonia, fibrosis)
- Patients with diagnosed Barrett's esophagus require regular screening endoscopy and biopsy to evaluate for the development of esophageal carcinoma

10. Peptic Ulcer Disease

Etiology/Pathophysiology

- Erosion and ulceration of the gastric or duodenal mucosa, occurring secondary to a disrupted balance between parietal cell acid production and generation of mucous (to coat and protect the mucosa) and bicarbonate (to buffer the acid)
- Most cases are caused by *Helicobacter pylori* (*H. pylori*) infection
- Duodenal ulcers are associated with excess acid secretion
  - Zollinger-Ellison syndrome is caused by a gastrin-secreting tumor (gastrinoma), which stimulates acid production
- Gastric ulcers are associated with mucosal breakdown in the stomach (e.g., stress, steroids, NSAIDs)
  - Cushing's ulcer: Stress ulcer in brain injured patients
  - Curling's ulcer: Stress ulcer in burn patients
- Bleeding may occur if the ulcer penetrates into a blood vessel
- Perforation may occur if the ulcer penetrates completely through all layers of the bowel wall

Differential Dx

- Ulcer symptoms
  - Gastritis
  - Gastric cancer
  - Pancreatic cancer
  - Cholelithiasis
  - Biliary dyskinesia
  - Pancreatitis
- Perforation symptoms
  - Ruptured colonic diverticulum
  - Appendicitis
  - Cholecystitis
  - Ischemic bowel
  - Ectopic pregnancy
  - Ruptured AAA

Presentation/Signs & Symptoms

- Gnawing/burning epigastric or right upper quadrant pain
  - Symptoms of gastric ulcers are exacerbated by eating
  - Symptoms of duodenal ulcers are decreased with meals but increased 2–3 hours after meals
- Indigestion and heartburn
- GI bleeding may occur, resulting in hematemesis, melena, anemia, and guaiac positive stools
- A perforated ulcer presents with immediate onset of severe pain and peritoneal signs
- *A perforated ulcer rarely bleeds and a bleeding ulcer rarely perforates*

Diagnostic Evaluation

- Upper GI endoscopy (EGD) is diagnostic
  - Offers direct visualization of the mucosa
  - Allows biopsy to evaluate for *H. pylori* infection and rule out cancer
  - May be therapeutic for a bleeding ulcer
- Upper GI series with barium swallow is less invasive and cheaper, but has lower sensitivity
- *H. pylori* serologic testing may be indicated
- CBC may reveal anemia due to chronic blood loss
- In cases of perforation, an upright chest X-ray will reveal free air under the diaphragm
  - EGD and UGI are contraindicated in suspected perforations
- For severe or recalcitrant disease, check gastrin level to screen for Zollinger-Ellison syndrome

Treatment/Management

- Eradicate *H. pylori* with triple therapy for 2 weeks (e.g., omeprazole, clarithromycin, and amoxicillin; bismuth, metronidazole, and tetracycline)
- Decrease or eliminate exacerbating factors, such as smoking, NSAIDs, and steroids
- Antacids, H2 blockers, proton pump inhibitors, and sulcralfate are sufficient therapy in most cases
- Perforation requires emergency surgical exploration
- Surgery may also be indicated in cases of failed medical therapy, intractable bleeding, gastric outlet obstruction, and Zollinger-Ellison syndrome
- Surgical interventions include oversewing of ulcer (for perforation or bleeding), pyloroplasty with vagotomy, antrectomy with vagotomy, or hemigastrectomy

Prognosis/Complications

- >85% cure rate with medical therapy alone
- Untreated ulcer disease may lead to gastric outlet obstruction due to chronic inflammation and scarring
- There is a risk of malignant transformation with gastric ulcers

11. Gastritis

Etiology/Pathophysiology

- Inflammation of the gastric mucosa
- Acute erosive gastritis: Self-limited irritation due to an irritant (e.g., NSAIDs, alcohol), severe physiologic stress (e.g., major surgery, burns, ventilator), or local trauma (e.g., NG tube)
- Chronic gastritis, type A: Inflammation of the proximal stomach due to pernicious anemia, atrophic gastritis, achlorhydria, autoimmune disease, or radiation
- Chronic gastritis, type B: Inflammation of the distal stomach or antrum due to *Helicobacter pylori* infection
- Reflux gastritis: Irritation due to the presence of bile and pancreatic juice in the stomach secondary to absent or non-functioning pylorus (e.g., following a partial gastrectomy)
- Hemorrhagic gastritis: Gastritis with significant hemorrhage as a reaction to severe stress (e.g., ICU patients, shock, hypoxia, ischemia, uremia)

Differential Dx

- Peptic ulcer disease
- GERD
- Gastroenteritis
- Gastric cancer
- Esophageal cancer
- Pancreatitis
- Biliary tract disease
- Myocardial infarction or coronary ischemia

Presentation/Signs & Symptoms

- Burning epigastric pain or discomfort that worsens with eating
- Dyspepsia
- Anorexia
- Nausea/vomiting
- Bleeding may be present, resulting in hematemesis, melena, and/or shock

Diagnostic Evaluation

- CBC will reveal microcytic anemia in chronic cases
- Upper GI endoscopy with biopsy is diagnostic
- *H. pylori* testing
- Check gastrin levels in patients who may have decreased acid production (chronic gastritis, type A) to rule out secondary hypergastrinemia (gastrin >1000 pg/mL)
- Rule out other potential causes of epigastric pain (e.g., pancreatitis, coronary disease)

Treatment/Management

- Reduce exposure to irritating agents
- Reduce acid production to protect the gastric mucosa with H2 blockers, proton pump inhibitor, and/or sucralfate
- Symptomatic *H. pylori* gastritis is treated with triple therapy for 2 weeks (e.g., omeprazole, clarithromycin, and amoxicillin; bismuth, metronidazole, and ampicillin/tetracycline)
- Antacid prophylaxis should be administered for most critically ill patients
- Severe bleeding in cases of stress gastritis may be treated endoscopically; in rare cases, unrelenting hemorrhage may require gastrectomy

Prognosis/Complications

- Acute gastritis generally heals within a few days
- Increased incidence of gastric ulcers and gastric cancer with chronic gastritis, type A
- Gastritis can be complicated by GI bleeding and recurrent symptoms

12. Gastric Cancer

Etiology/Pathophysiology

- Nearly 95% of cases are adenocarcinoma (5% are lymphoma; sarcoma and carcinoid are rare)
  - Intestinal type is most common type: Grows as a discrete tumor and eventually erodes through stomach wall to nearby organs
  - Diffuse type: A poorly differentiated cancer that has little cell cohesion; thus, it grows outward along the submucosa of the stomach and widely envelopes the stomach without producing a discrete mass formation (i.e., "linitis plastica")
- Risk factors include *Helicobacter pylori* infection, chronic gastritis (atrophic gastritis, pernicious anemia), history of partial gastrectomy, diets high in nitrites, salted, smoked, or poorly preserved foods, diets low in fruits and vegetables, alcohol, smoking
- Usually a disease of older patients
- Adenomatous polyps and chronic gastric ulcers have a risk of malignant transformation
- 40% occur in the antrum; 30% in the body and fundus
- Decreasing in frequency over the past century; previously the #1 cancer in U.S. and worldwide—now #2 worldwide and #11 in U.S.

Differential Dx

- Gastritis
- Peptic ulcer disease
- Esophageal cancer
- Pancreatic cancer
- Amyloidosis
- Sarcoidosis
- Peutz-Jeghers syndrome
- Polyps (hyperplastic, adenomatous, or inflammatory)
- Carcinoid

Presentation/Signs & Symptoms

- Early tumors tend to be asymptomatic
- Weight loss, early satiety, and pain are the most frequent symptoms
- Nausea and vomiting
- Dysphagia and/or anorexia
- Melena or occult hemorrhage
- Abdominal mass may be palpable in advanced cases
- Ascites
- Blumer's shelf may be found on rectal exam (metastatic disease to the anterior rectal wall)
- Virchow's node (left supraclavicular metastasis), Krukenberg's tumor (ovarian metastasis), or Sister Mary Joseph node (periumbilical metastases) may be present

Diagnostic Evaluation

- Upper GI endoscopy with biopsy is diagnostic
- Upper GI series may show ulcer, mass, or distortion of the stomach; however, biopsy is usually required
- CBC may show iron deficiency anemia
- CT scan and endoscopic ultrasound are used to evaluate for metastatic disease and for staging
- Staging laparoscopy or laparotomy may be used to evaluate for metastatic disease

Treatment/Management

- Complete resection with wide margins presents the only hope for cure
  - Total gastrectomy for proximal lesions (body, cardia, fundus)
  - Subtotal gastrectomy for distal lesions (pylorus, antrum)
  - If adjacent organs are involved (e.g., spleen, tail of pancreas, colon, omentum, distal esophagus, duodenum), they may be resected with gastric resection
- Incurable cases may be palliated by surgery, chemotherapy, or radiation to relieve symptoms
- Gastric lymphoma can be treated with radiation or chemotherapy

Prognosis/Complications

- Disease is usually advanced upon diagnosis
- If distant metastases, lymph node metastases, or involvement of adjacent organs are noted, prognosis is extremely poor
- Average 5-year survival in U.S. <20%
- Average 5-year survival in Japan is nearly 50% due to aggressive screening (upper GI endoscopy with biopsy) and early surgical resection

13. Zollinger-Ellison Syndrome

Etiology/Pathophysiology

- A syndrome of recurrent, refractory ulcers and diarrhea caused by a gastrin-secreting tumor (gastrinoma)
  - 90% of gastrinomas occur in the "ZE triangle," formed by the porta hepatis (junction of the cystic duct and common bile duct), head of the pancreas, and the mid-duodenum
  - The most common sites of gastrinomas are the pancreas and duodenum; the remainder of cases occurs in the stomach, lymph nodes, or spleen
- The autonomous gastrin secretion causes maximal parietal cell acid production, eventually leading to severe ulcer disease
- Nearly 80% of cases are sporadic
- About 25% of cases occur as part of MEN-I syndrome (60% of MEN-I patients develop pancreatic tumors; about 50% of these tumors are gastrinomas)
- About half of gastrinomas are malignant, with metastases most commonly occurring to the liver

Differential Dx

- Peptic ulcer disease
- Elevated gastrin states
  - Chronic gastritis
  - Pernicious anemia
  - Post-vagotomy
  - Renal failure
  - Short gut syndrome
  - Gastric outlet obstruction
  - Gastric cancer
  - *Helicobacter pylori* infection
- MEN-I syndrome (parathyroid hyperplasia, pancreatic tumors, and pituitary tumors)

Presentation/Signs & Symptoms

- Abdominal pain (usually epigastric)
- Recurrent or recalcitrant peptic ulcer disease
- Diarrhea and/or steatorrhea
- Esophagitis
- Dysphagia
- Recalcitrant emesis
- Weight loss
- Patients with MEN-I syndrome may also present with hyperparathyroidism (e.g., signs of hypercalcemia, nephrolithiasis) and pituitary tumors (e.g., headache, visual disturbances)

Diagnostic Evaluation

- Elevated serum gastrin
  - Serum gastrin >200 pg/mL suggests the diagnosis
  - Serum gastrin >1000 pg/mL is diagnostic
- Gastric acid analysis to confirm elevated production
- Secretin stimulation test reveals a paradoxical increase in gastrin levels upon secretin administration
- Endoscopy will reveal evidence of peptic ulcer disease
- Measure serum calcium, cortisol, and prolactin to rule out MEN-I syndrome
- CT, MRI, radionucleotide scan, endoscopic ultrasound, or intra-operative ultrasound may localize the tumor
- Selective arterial secretin stimulation if the above tests fail
- If the tumor is metastatic or unresectable, percutaneous or laparoscopic biopsy may be used to confirm the diagnosis

Treatment/Management

- Surgical resection should be attempted
  - Localization and excision of the tumor
  - Pancreaticoduodenectomy may be necessary for larger tumors around the duodenum
  - Liver metastases should be resected if possible
- Proton pump inhibitors (e.g., omeprazole) should be administered to control acid secretion while planning surgery and for unresectable tumors
- Chemotherapy for widely metastatic or incurable disease may include streptozotocin, 5-flurouracil, or doxorubicin
- Failure of medical treatment may necessitate total gastrectomy

Prognosis/Complications

- 70% overall 5-year survival
- 35% of tumors are resectable
- 35% 5-year survival in patients with metastatic disease upon initial presentation

14. Carcinoid Tumors

Etiology/Pathophysiology

- A neuroendocrine tumor classified as an APUD (amine precursor uptake and decarboxylation) tumor—also called "APUDoma"
  - 80% arise in the GI tract (most commonly in the appendix and terminal ileum)
  - 25% of all small bowel tumors (small bowel carcinoids are multiple in about one-third of cases)
  - 10% occur in the lungs
  - Other sites (e.g., kidney, pancreas, testicles, ovaries) are less common
- May be associated with MEN-I syndrome, Crohn's disease, or Gardner syndrome
- Systemic "carcinoid syndrome" occurs in about 20% of cases due to release of serotonin and other vasoactive compounds from the tumor
  - Symptoms are often brought on by stress or alcohol
  - Carcinoid syndrome usually only occurs when there is liver metastases

Differential Dx

- Other small bowel tumors
  - Adenoma
  - GIST (GI stromal tumor)
  - Lipoma
  - Adenocarcinoma
  - Lymphoma
- Other causes of abdominal pain
  - Appendicitis
  - Gastritis
  - Mesenteric ischemia
  - Gallbladder disease
- Other causes of bowel obstruction
  - Adhesions
  - Hernia

Presentation/Signs & Symptoms

- Most cases are asymptomatic
- Appendiceal carcinoids often present as appendicitis due to obstruction of the appendiceal lumen by the tumor
- Bowel obstruction
- Intussusception
- Carcinoid syndrome results in flushing, cyanosis, tachycardia, diarrhea, bronchospasm, edema, ascites, and hypotension

Diagnostic Evaluation

- Often found incidentally during appendectomy
- Confirm diagnosis by measuring for 24-hour urine for 5-HIAA levels, which are breakdown products of serotonin
- Abdominal CT scan may be helpful to delineate extent of disease, multifocal involvement, and metastases

Treatment/Management

- Resection is generally the treatment-of-choice
  - For appendiceal carcinoid <1.5 cm in diameter, appendectomy is considered curative
  - For appendiceal carcinoid >1.5 cm in diameter, right hemicolectomy is indicated
  - Pulmonary carcinoid is best treated by resection
- Chemotherapy may be used for metastatic disease
- Debulking of hepatic metastases via surgery, radiofrequency ablation, or chemo-embolization may relieve carcinoid syndrome
- Octreotide may be used symptomatically to block the release of vasoactive compounds from the tumor

Prognosis/Complications

- Appendiceal carcinoid tumors are usually discovered early in the course of disease
- Resection is curative for most cases of appendiceal carcinoid; however, 4% will metastasize to the liver
- Carcinoid tumors that arise outside the appendix have usually spread locally or metastasized at the time of diagnosis
- Pulmonary carcinoid has excellent prognosis

15. Small Bowel Tumors

Etiology/Pathophysiology

- Benign small bowel tumors include GIST (gastrointestinal stromal tumor), lipoma, adenoma, hamartoma, and hemangioma
- Malignant tumors include adenocarcinoma, carcinoid, lymphoma, and GISS (gastrointestinal stromal sarcoma)
- These tumors are fairly uncommon, perhaps due to the alkaline fluid in the small bowel or because the rapid transit time through small bowel reduces exposure to carcinogens
- Associated with Crohn's disease and familial adenomatous polyposis
- Immunosuppressed patients are at greater risk
- See also "Carcinoid Tumors" entry for further discussion

Differential Dx

- Neurofibroma
- Metastatic disease (e.g., breast, colon, melanoma)
- Causes of small bowel obstruction (e.g., adhesions, hernia, foreign bodies)

Presentation/Signs & Symptoms

- Most cases are asymptomatic
- Abdominal pain
- GI bleeding
- Weight loss
- Abdominal mass
- Symptoms of small bowel obstruction (e.g., nausea, vomiting, distension)

Diagnostic Evaluation

- CBC may reveal microcytic anemia
- Imaging studies are fairly non-sensitive for small bowel tumors
    - Small bowel follow-through study
    - Enteroclysis study (allows detailed examination of the small bowel mucosa)
    - Abdominal CT scan may reveal larger tumors
- Enteroscopy through the ileocecal valve (per rectum) or beyond the Ligament of Treitz (per orum) may be attempted but is difficult
- In actively bleeding tumors, angiography may be useful to localize the tumor

Treatment/Management

- Resection is the treatment of choice for malignant or symptomatic tumors
- Chemotherapy may be useful in some cases

Prognosis/Complications

- These tumors are frequently diagnosed late in the course of disease due to the non-specific presentation
- Prognosis varies upon pathology

16. Small Bowel Obstruction

Etiology/Pathophysiology

- Partial or complete blockage of the small intestine
- The most common causes of small bowel obstruction are adhesions, hernias, and tumors
  - Other causes of small bowel obstruction include foreign bodies (e.g., gallstone ileus), intussusception, inflammation (e.g., Crohn's disease, radiation enteritis), and volvulus (bowel twists around on itself)
- Increased intraluminal pressure causes wall dilatation, decreased absorption, and third-spacing of fluid into the bowel lumen and wall; this results in volume depletion, hypotension, and possibly translocation of bacteria into the systemic circulation with ensuing sepsis
- Strangulation may occur if the blood supply becomes compromised, resulting in bowel ischemia, necrosis, and perforation
- May be a closed- or open-loop obstruction
  - Closed-loop obstructions have no outlet (proximally or distally), so complications occur rapidly (especially strangulation)
  - Open-loop obstruction may transiently decompress by emesis, so progression of complications occurs slower

Differential Dx

- Large bowel obstruction
- Ileus
- Gastroenteritis
- Pseudo-obstruction (a chronic disorder of intestinal motility due to collagen vascular disease, diabetes, or drugs)
- Appendicitis
- Mesenteric ischemia
- Pancreatitis
- Cholecystitis
- Pelvic inflammatory disease

Presentation/Signs & Symptoms

- Colicky abdominal pain
- Vomiting
  - The more frequent the emesis, the more proximal the obstruction
  - May not occur in a closed-loop obstruction
- Bowel movements and flatus may be decreased or absent
- High pitched bowel sounds
- Borborygmi
- Abdominal distention and tenderness
- Peritoneal signs are present if strangulation or perforation occurs

Diagnostic Evaluation

- History and physical exam (including search for hernias and history of prior abdominal surgery)
- CBC will reveal leukocytosis (marked leukocytosis in cases of strangulation)
- Amylase may be slightly elevated
- Plain films may reveal a distended bowel, air-fluid levels, stair-stepping, free-air (if perforation occurs), foreign body, or absence of gas in the rectum
- CT scan with oral contrast may show "transition-zone" from dilated, obstructed bowel to normal, collapsed bowel
- Barium enema contrast study may be used to rule out large bowel obstructions and differentiate mechanical obstruction from ileus

Treatment/Management

- Conservative treatment with nasogastric suction and aggressive IV fluid resuscitation may be sufficient for non-complete obstructions
- Surgical intervention is indicated for complete obstructions, failure of conservative therapy, or signs of strangulation
- Surgical treatment is directed at the underlying etiology of the obstruction
  - Lysis of adhesions
  - Repair of hernia
  - Removal of foreign body
  - Resection of intussuscepted bowel
  - Resection or bypass of malignant obstructions

Prognosis/Complications

- Strangulated bowel can become necrotic and gangrenous in as little as 6 hours—accurate and quick diagnosis is essential
- Delayed diagnosis of closed-loop obstruction or strangulation worsens the prognosis
- Mortality increases dramatically (from 10–50% to 50%) if bowel ischemia is present at the time of operation
- Obstruction secondary to adhesions will recur in 20% of patients
- Obstructions secondary to gallstones will recur in nearly 10% of patients, unless the gallbladder is removed
- Many open-loop obstructions will resolve with conservative treatment

17. Large Bowel Obstruction

Etiology/Pathophysiology

- Partial or complete blockage of the colon
- The most common cause of large bowel obstruction is colon or rectal cancer
  - Less common causes include volvulus, diverticulitis, hernia, fecal impaction, intussusception, ischemic colitis, radiation injury, endometriosis, and foreign bodies
- Obstruction may be difficult to distinguish from motility disorders
- Colonic pseudo-obstruction (Ogilvie's syndrome) is a paralytic ileus of the large bowel
  - Associated factors for the development of pseudo-obstruction include increasing age, postoperative ileus (especially after orthopedic and cardiac procedures), trauma, bedrest, heavy narcotic use, electrolyte imbalance, dementia, drugs with anti-motility effect, alcoholism

Differential Dx

- Small bowel obstruction
- Severe constipation
- Motility dysfunction (e.g., ileus, Ogilvie's syndrome, colonic inertia)

Presentation/Signs & Symptoms

- Colicky abdominal pain and distention
- Failure to pass feces or flatus
- Feculent emesis if the ileocecal valve is incompetent
- Diarrhea may be present despite the obstruction
- Weight loss and change in caliber of stools should raise the suspicion of colon or rectal carcinoma

Diagnostic Evaluation

- Flat and upright abdominal films are often diagnostic, showing dilated bowel proximal to the obstruction and absence of gas distal to the obstruction
- Abdominal CT may be used if plain films are unclear to locate the obstruction and demonstrate the obstructing lesion (e.g., colon tumor, diverticulitis)
- Labs should include CBC, electrolytes, and renal function
- Gastrograffin enema may be used to differentiate between pseudo-obstruction and mechanical obstruction
- Colonoscopy may be used to identify and biopsy colon lesions and may decompress the obstruction; however, should not be used if diverticulitis is suspected

Treatment/Management

- Nasogastric tube decompression
- IV fluids administration
- Indications for emergent surgical intervention include free-air (indicating perforation) and increasing cecal diameter (>15 cm usually results in perforation; >10 cm is a concern for perforation)
  - Proximal and transverse colon obstructions require right hemicolectomy with ileocolic anastomosis +/− ileostomy
  - Left-sided obstructions require resection with diverting colostomy or ileostomy
  - Obstructions due to rectal cancer require diverting colostomy and neoadjuvant therapy; primary resection is usually delayed
  - Sigmoid volvulus requires decompression with sigmoidoscopy followed by resection
- Colonic pseudo-obstruction may be treated with colonoscopic decompression

Prognosis/Complications

- 20% mortality rate
- Mortality increases dramatically if ischemia or perforation occurs
- Cancer patients presenting with obstruction at the time of diagnosis have a worse prognosis
- Complications of surgery include abscess, bleeding, fistula formation, or anastomotic leak

18. Appendicitis

Etiology/Pathophysiology

- Appendicitis is the most common abdominal surgical emergency
- 10% of the U.S. population will develop appendicitis at some time
- Luminal obstruction is thought to be the inciting event leading to inflammation and infection of the appendix
  - Obstruction is most commonly caused by a fecalith, which results from accumulation and inspissation of fecal matter around vegetable fibers
  - Other potential causes of lumen obstruction include neoplasm, foreign objects, and enlarged lymphoid follicles
- Obstruction of the lumen leads to distention, increased intraluminal pressure, venous engorgement, impaired arterial blood supply, and ischemia
- As the ischemic mucosal barrier breaks down, bacterial invasion from the colon occurs, resulting in inflammation, necrosis, and rupture
- Histologically, obstruction is identified in only 30–40% of cases; potential causes in the absence of luminal obstruction include mucosal ulceration secondary to infection (e.g., *Yersinia*, virus)

Differential Dx

- Gastroenteritis
- Perforated peptic ulcer
- Meckel's diverticulitis
- Acute cholecystitis
- Mesenteric lymphadenitis
- Intestinal obstruction
- Crohn's disease
- Ileitis
- Diverticulitis
- Renal colic
- Ectopic pregnancy
- Ruptured ovarian follicle
- Pelvic inflammatory disease
- Tubo-ovarian abscess
- Mittelschmertz

Presentation/Signs & Symptoms

- Vague, periumbilical or epigastric pain that migrates to the right lower quadrant (McBurney's point)
- Low fever, anorexia, nausea/vomiting
- Atypical findings are often found in children, the elderly, and in patients with a retrocecal appendix
- High fevers and rebound tenderness suggests a ruptured appendix
- Rovsing's sign (referred rebound tenderness): Right lower quadrant (RLQ) pain caused by palpation of the left lower quadrant
- Psoas sign: RLQ pain upon passive extension of right leg
- Obturator sign: RLQ pain upon passive internal rotation of flexed leg

Diagnostic Evaluation

- History and physical exam generally suggests the diagnosis
- CBC generally reveals mild leukocytosis; however, a normal CBC does not rule out appendicitis
- Urine hCG test is necessary in all females of reproductive age to rule out pregnancy; however, a positive pregnancy test does not rule out appendicitis
- Abdominal and pelvic CT scans with contrast is especially useful to workup patients with atypical presentations (e.g., retrocecal appendix), to rule out pelvic pathology in premenopausal females (e.g., ectopic pregnancy, ruptured ovarian cyst), and to rule out appendiceal abscess
- Ultrasound is diagnostic if positive but does not rule out appendicitis if negative
- Abdominal X-rays are usually not required but may show a fecalith in the RLQ

Treatment/Management

- Appendectomy (laparoscopic or open) is the treatment of choice
  - Emergent surgery is generally required, as rupture can occur within 24 hours of symptom onset
  - Diagnostic laparoscopy with or without appendectomy can be used in patients with atypical presentations or to rule out pelvic pathology
  - Administer peri-operative IV antibiotics against enteric organisms (gram negatives, anaerobes, and *Enterococcus*), such as a third generation cephalosporin and metronidazole
- Pre-operative identification of an appendiceal abscess may be treated by percutaneous drainage (CT- or ultrasound-guided) and IV antibiotics, with an elective appendectomy several months later (interval appendectomy)

Prognosis/Complications

- Rapid recovery and low mortality with early diagnosis and treatment
- Rupture, abscess formation, and/or peritonitis complicate treatment; repeat operations and long recovery may follow

19. Diverticular Disease of the Colon

Etiology/Pathophysiology

- Diverticulosis: Acquired disease of the colon caused by outpouchings of the colonic mucosa and submucosa through the muscularis layer; this herniation occurs at sites where intramural blood vessels penetrate the muscular layer
- Common in industrialized countries with diets low in fiber
- A disease of advancing age (half the U.S. population is affected by age 60; nearly all people over age 80 are affected)
- Associated with low fiber diet →↓ bulk of stool →↑ pressure generated by colonic peristalsis → herniations at focal weaknesses in colon wall
  - Diverticula may be present anywhere in the colon (most commonly in the sigmoid)
- Diverticulosis itself is asymptomatic; however, complications include infection (diverticulitis) and bleeding (diverticular hemorrhage)
  - Diverticulitis (*without bleeding*) occurs in 20% of patients with diverticulosis: Infection and inflammation of a colonic diverticulum
  - Diverticular hemorrhage (*without infection*) is the most common cause of lower GI bleeding in the elderly

Differential Dx

- Diverticulitis
  - Appendicitis
  - Colon cancer
  - Gastroenteritis
  - Bowel obstruction
  - Irritable bowel syndrome
  - Infectious colitis (e.g., *Clostridium difficile, Yersinia*)
  - Ulcerative colitis
  - Crohn's disease
  - Pelvic cancer
- Diverticular hemorrhage
  - Upper GI bleeding
  - Arteriovenous malformation
  - Infectious colitis (e.g., *C. difficile, Yersinia*)
  - Polyps

Presentation/Signs & Symptoms

- Diverticulosis is usually asymptomatic
  - Patient may give a history of mild lower abdominal pain with constipation and/or diarrhea, often relieved by bowel movements
- Diverticulitis presents with fever, left lower quadrant pain and tenderness
  - Nausea, vomiting, diarrhea, and dysuria may be present
  - Inflammatory mass in the left lower quadrant may be palpated (phlegmon)
  - Peritoneal signs indicate perforation
  - Bleeding does not occur
- Diverticular hemorrhage is painless and completely asymptomatic
  - Sudden onset of significant bleeding per rectum

Diagnostic Evaluation

- Asymptomatic diverticulosis is often incidentally identified on colonoscopy, abdominal CT scan, or barium enema
- Diverticulitis is a clinical diagnosis with a triad of left lower quadrant pain, fever, and leukocytosis
  - Abdominal CT scan is the diagnostic test of choice; reveals bowel wall thickening, pericolic inflammation, and possibly abscess formation
  - Barium enema and colonoscopy are contraindicated in acute diverticulitis as they may increase the risk of perforation
- Diverticular hemorrhage
  - Rule out upper GI bleeding by nasogastric tube placement and/or upper GI endoscopy
  - Colonoscopy to identify site of bleeding and confirm diverticula
  - If colonoscopy cannot reveal the site of active bleeding, consider mesenteric angiography

Treatment/Management

- Uncomplicated diverticulitis is treated with bowel rest (no oral intake) and IV antibiotics (e.g., third generation cephalosporin and metronidazole)
  - Elective sigmoid resection is indicated after the second episode of diverticulitis
- Complicated diverticulitis is abscess or fistula formation, frank perforation, or bowel obstruction
  - Abscess is treated with percutaneous drainage (CT- or ultrasound-guided) and antibiotics
  - Perforation requires emergent laparotomy with sigmoid resection, colostomy formation, and mucous fistula of rectum (Hartmann's procedure)
  - Fistula formation and bowel obstruction require resection and possible temporary colostomy
- Diverticular hemorrhage requires fluid resuscitation
  - Resection is indicated in severe or recurrent bleeding
  - See "Lower GI Bleeding" entry

Prognosis/Complications

- Patients with diverticulosis require fiber supplementation (high fiber diet or psyllium)
- Complications of diverticulitis include perforation, fistula (to bladder, vagina, or skin), abscess formation, and sepsis
- Patients with acute diverticulitis have a 40% risk of recurrence and 80% risk of recurrence following the second episode; thus, elective resection is indicated after the second episode and in young patients after the initial episode
  - In patients >50, follow-up with a colonoscopy after the acute event resolves in order to rule out cancer
- Patients with diverticular hemorrhage have a 40% risk of rebleeding after the first episode and 90% risk of rebleeding after the second episode; thus, elective resection may be indicated

20. Crohn's Disease

Etiology/Pathophysiology

- A chronic, relapsing-remitting, inflammatory condition with flare-ups secondary to stress, infections, NSAIDs, and medication noncompliance
- May affect any part of Gl tract from mouth to anus
  - Primarily affects the ileum
  - 20% colon only, 33% ileum only, 45% colon and ileum, 2% rest of GI tract (e.g., duodenum, esophagus, mouth)
  - Usually spares the rectum
- Characteristic histologic findings
  - Transmural (full-thickness) inflammation of the involved bowel
  - Normal bowel alternates with areas of disease ("skip lesions" or "cobblestoning")
  - Granulomas (non-caseating) are present in one-third of cases
  - Perforation, stricture, and fistula formation may occur
- Bimodal incidence: 20–30s is the most common onset of disease; also common in patients >50
- Female > male

Differential Dx

- Ulcerative colitis
- Bacterial diarrhea (e.g., *Shigella, Salmonella, Campylobacter, Yersinia, E. coli*)
- Parasitic or viral GI disease
- *Clostridium difficile* colitis
- Appendicitis
- Diverticulitis
- Mesenteric ischemia
- Colon cancer
- Irritable bowel syndrome
- Pelvic inflammatory disease
- Endometriosis
- Radiation colitis
- Collagen vascular disease

Presentation/Signs & Symptoms

- Diarrhea
- Abdominal pain (colicky)
- Weight loss
- Fever
- RLQ mass (may mimic appendicitis) and steatorrhea may be present if there is extensive ileal involvement
- Symptoms of complications may be present
  - Bowel obstruction
  - Fistula formation
  - Intra-abdominal abscess
  - Perianal or perirectal disease
  - Peritonitis, shock, and/or sepsis may occur with perforation

Diagnostic Evaluation

- Definitive diagnosis of Crohn's is made by colonoscopy, upper GI series with small bowel follow-through, and barium enema
  - Nodularity, rigidity, cobblestoning, fistulas, and strictures may be seen
- Check stool cultures for bacteria and ova/parasites
- Fecal leukocytes will be present in stool analysis
- Abdominal X-rays may show perforation (free-air) or obstruction
- Abdominal CT may show free-air, abscesses, thickened bowel loops or mesentery, and fistula formation
- CBC may reveal anemia and leukocytosis

Treatment/Management

- IV fluids as necessary to correct dehydration
- NG tube insertion and no oral intake may be necessary in acute flare-ups or bowel obstruction
- Antidiarrheal therapy (e.g., loperamide)
- Acute disease is treated with aminosalicylates, antibiotics (metronidazole or ciprofloxacin), and immunosuppressants
- Infliximab (TNF-α inhibitor) may be useful in acute flare-ups and possibly as a maintenance therapy
- Steroids, azathioprine, and 6-MP are often used in moderate to severe cases
- Ileal and/or colon resection may be useful; however, disease tends to recur around areas of surgery
  - 50% of patients require further surgery within 5 years

Prognosis/Complications

- High recurrence rate
- Complications include perforation, abscess, obstruction, fistula (to bowel, bladder, or vagina), perianal fissures/abscesses, malabsorption syndromes, and cancer (colon and small bowel)
- Involvement of other organ symptoms occurs in 10% of patients, including joints (enteropathic arthropathy), skin (erythema nodosum), eye (uveitis, iritis), liver (cholelithiasis, primary sclerosing cholangitis, pancreatitis), pulmonary embolus, and bone (osteoporosis)
- Patients require regular screening colonoscopy

21. Ulcerative Colitis

Etiology/Pathophysiology

- A chronic, relapsing-remitting, inflammatory condition involving mucosa and submucosa of the rectum and colon
  - Rectum is always involved
  - The remainder of the upper GI tract is spared
  - 80% of patients present with segmental colitis; 20% present with pancolitis
- Characteristic histologic findings
  - Involves only the mucosa and submucosa (not full-thickness)
  - Diffuse, continuous mucosal inflammation (no skip areas)
  - No small bowel involvement
  - Crypt abscesses are formed but no granuloma formation or fistulas
- Male > female
- Family history is important: 10 times greater risk in first-degree relatives
- Bimodal peak at ages 20–35 and 50–65
- Higher incidence than Crohn's disease

Differential Dx

- Crohn's disease
- Bacterial diarrhea (*Shigella, Salmonella, Campylobacter, Yersinia, E. coli*)
- Parasitic or viral GI disease
- *Clostridium difficile* colitis
- Appendicitis
- Diverticulitis
- Mesenteric ischemia
- Colon cancer
- Irritable bowel syndrome
- Pelvic inflammatory disease
- Endometriosis
- Radiation colitis
- Collagen vascular disease

Presentation/Signs & Symptoms

- Bloody diarrhea with periods of constipation
- Lower abdominal pain and cramps
- Weight loss
- Fever
- 15% present with a fulminant course (e.g., sepsis, toxic megacolon, perforation)
- Tenesmus (sensation of fullness in the rectum)

Diagnostic Evaluation

- Definitive diagnosis is made by colonoscopy with biopsy, revealing continuous inflammation with friability, exudates, and polyps
- Flexible sigmoidoscopy is 90–95% accurate if the rectum and distal colon are involved
- Check stool cultures for bacteria and ova/parasites
- Fecal leukocytes will be present in stool analysis
- Abdominal X-rays may show perforation (free-air) or obstruction
- Abdominal CT may show free-air, abscesses, or toxic megacolon

Treatment/Management

- IV fluids, bowel rest (NG tube and no oral intake) may be necessary in acute flare-ups or obstruction
- Antidiarrheal therapy (e.g., loperamide)
- Acute disease is treated with aminosalicylates (e.g., sulfasalazine, mesalamine) given orally or by enema
- Immunosuppressants are added for moderate to severe disease (glucocorticoids, azathioprine, 6-MP)
- Surgical intervention is necessary for unrelenting hemorrhage, toxic megacolon, failure of medical therapy, obstruction, suspicion of malignancy, systemic complications, children who fail to thrive, or longstanding disease
  - Surgical options include total proctocolectomy with J-pouch and ileoanal anastomosis, total proctocolectomy with permanent end ileostomy, total proctocolectomy with continent ileostomy
  - Surveillance for cancer is necessary if any part of rectum remains (e.g., J-pouch)

Prognosis/Complications

- Risk of colon cancer becomes significant after 10 years
- Complications include colorectal cancer, perforation, toxic megacolon, and obstruction
- Complications of surgery include bleeding, infection (e.g., abscess), pouch dysfunction, bowel obstruction, and autonomic nerve damage leading to sexual dysfunction
- Involvement of other organ symptoms occurs in 10% of patients, including joints (enteropathic arthropathy), skin (erythema nodosum), eye (uveitis, iritis), liver (cholelithiasis, primary sclerosing cholangitis, pancreatitis), pulmonary embolus, and bone (osteoporosis)
- Patients require regular screening colonoscopy, unless the entire colon and rectum have been removed

22. Colon Cancer

Etiology/Pathophysiology

- Colon cancer is the most common visceral cancer and the third most common cause of cancer death in males and females; incidence increases with age
- 95% of cases are adenocarcinoma
- Thought to arise from neoplastic polyps ("polyp-cancer sequence")
    - High risk polyps tend to be >2 cm, villous, and sessile
- Risk factors include hereditary syndromes (e.g., Lynch syndrome, familial polyposis syndromes), high fat diets, low fiber diets, inflammatory bowel disease, radiation, and history of ureterocolostomy
- 5–10% have synchronous lesions (two simultaneous colonic sites of cancer); 20% develop metachronous lesions (later development of cancer at a another colonic site)
- 15–20% present with metastatic disease
    - Liver is the most common site of distant metastases
    - Lung is the most common site of metastases for rectal cancer

Differential Dx

- Benign stricture
- Benign polyp
- Diverticulitis
- Ulcerative colitis
- Crohn's disease
- Pelvic cancer
- Pelvic inflammatory disease
- Ischemic colitis

Presentation/Signs & Symptoms

- Weight loss, fatigue, and weakness
- Change in bowel habits and caliber of stool
- Right-sided cancers present with right-sided mass, iron deficiency anemia, postprandial discomfort, and occult heme-positive stools
- Left-sided cancers present with alternating diarrhea and constipation, increased risk of obstruction, and hematochezia
- Signs of obstruction may be present (e.g., nausea/vomiting, no bowel movements or flatus, abdominal distension)
- Rectal carcinoma presents with palpable mass on rectal exam and tenesmus (sensation of rectal fullness)

Diagnostic Evaluation

- Microcytic anemia with guaiac-positive stools should prompt evaluation for colon cancer
- Colonoscopy with biopsy is diagnostic and may allow for removal of early lesions
- Barium enema may detect polyps and cancer but is not as sensitive as colonoscopy
- CT scan is necessary for staging and to search for metastases
- Colonic tumor markers (e.g., CEA, CA-125) should be drawn on all colon cancer patients prior to treatment to be used to follow disease recurrence
- Metastatic workup should include LFTs and CT of the thorax, abdomen, and pelvis

Treatment/Management

- Surgical resection is curative for early cancers (stages I and II)
- Surgical resection plus adjuvant chemotherapy (5-fluorouracil and leucovorin) is indicated for some stage II lesions and stages III and IV lesions
- Treatment options for rectal carcinoma
    - Transrectal excision is an option for small lesions below the peritoneal reflection (T1 and some T2 lesions)
    - Neoadjuvant (pre-operative) therapy is indicated for locally advanced bulky tumors; improves sphincter preservation
    - Radiation and chemotherapy are mainstays of treatment
- Liver metastases may be resected, chemo-embolized, or direct arterial infusion chemotherapy into the hepatic artery

Prognosis/Complications

- Earlier staging was done by Duke's classification; however, TNM system is now most commonly used
- Quick TNM staging
    - Stage I: Any T1 or T2 lesion and N0
    - Stage II: Any T3 or T4 lesions and N0
    - Stage III: Any T with positive nodes
    - Stage IV: Metastatic disease (often involves the liver)
- 5-year survival by stage
    - Stage I: 80%
    - Stage II: 60%
    - Stage III: 30%
    - Stage IV: 5%
- Follow-up after resection should include regular colonic tumor marker levels, stool guaiac every 6 months, and colonoscopy every year

23. Anal Fissure

Etiology/Pathophysiology

- Anal fissure is a common and painful disorder that is often mistaken for hemorrhoids
- Most common cause of anal pain
- Begins as a crack or tear in the vertical axis of the squamous lining of the anal canal
- Caused by chronic constipation; the passage of hard stools tears the anal epithelium
- May be associated with a hyperactive anal sphincter or Crohn's disease

Differential Dx

- Hemorrhoids
- Anal cancer
- Ulcerative proctitis
- Fissures in non-midline locations should raise suspicion for Crohn's disease, syphilitic chancre, tuberculosis, or blood dyscrasias

Presentation/Signs & Symptoms

- Presents as a small midline longitudinal ulcer or tear at the dentate line
    - 90–95% are seen in the posterior midline; 5–10% are seen anteriorly
    - External skin tag often seen at the anal verge (sentinel pile)
- Pain with defecation
- Extremely painful rectal exam
- Frequently associated with a tight or stenotic anus

Diagnostic Evaluation

- Inspection
- Palpation
- Anoscopic exam
- If an underlying disease process is suspected, consider stool cultures, viral titers, serologies, and/or biopsy

Treatment/Management

- Conservative management is sufficient in 80–90% of cases
    - Sitz bath
    - Appropriate anal hygiene
    - High fiber diet and stool softeners
    - Nitroglycerin
    - Botulinum toxin injection
    - Calcium channel blockers
- Operative management with lateral internal sphincterotomy is the most effective treatment for chronic fissures
- Contraindicated in the presence of abscess or fistula

Prognosis/Complications

- Most fissures resolve with medical therapy alone
- Complications of surgery include abscess or fistula formation, bleeding, urinary retention, and fecal incontinence

24. Anal Fistula

Etiology/Pathophysiology

- The development of an abnormal communication (fistula) between the rectum and the perianal skin
- Develops following an infection of the anal crypts/glands with abscess formation (perirectal abscess) with ultimate erosion through to the perianal skin
- Often suspected with recurrent perirectal abscesses (especially if always in the same location)

Differential Dx

- Perirectal abscess
- Rectovaginal fistula
- Crohn's disease
- Tuberculosis
- Anal cancer
- Pilonidal abscess

Presentation/Signs & Symptoms

- Perianal drainage
- Recurrent perirectal abscesses
- Pain, excoriation, and itching

Diagnostic Evaluation

- Workup should include anoscopy to identify the internal opening and proctosigmoidoscopy to rule out inflammatory bowel disease
- Fistulography, endorectal ultrasound, or CT may be required in atypical, recurrent cases
- Goodsall's rule
  - Fistulas on the anterior aspect of the anus have direct communication to the rectum
  - Fistulas on the posterior aspect of the anus have curved tracts that converge to the posterior midline of the anal canal

Treatment/Management

- Most simple fistulas are treated surgically by fistulotomy (opening of the fistula tract)
- If the fistula appears to involve the sphincter, delayed sphincterotomy with seton (suture placed through fistula tract) insertion is necessary to allow the fistula to heal while maintaining sphincter integrity

Prognosis/Complications

- Complications of surgery include bleeding, infection, fecal incontinence, and anal stricture

25. Hemorrhoids

Etiology/Pathophysiology

- Results from engorgement of the venous plexus of the rectum/anus, with protrusion of mucosa
- The dentate line defines the junction of the rectum (columnar epithelium) with the anus (squamous epithelium)
    - External hemorrhoids occur below the dentate line
    - Internal hemorrhoids occur above the dentate line
- Location of hemorrhoids (hemorrhoid quadrants) occur in the right anterolateral quadrant of the anus, the right posterolateral quadrant, and the left lateral quadrant
- Risk factors include constipation, straining, portal hypertension, and pregnancy
- Classified by degree of prolapse
    - First-degree hemorrhoids do not prolapse
    - Second-degree hemorrhoids prolapse with defecation but spontaneously reduce
    - Third-degree hemorrhoids prolapse but require manual reduction
    - Fourth-degree hemorrhoids are prolapsed and cannot be reduced

Differential Dx

- Cancer
- Skin tag
- Rectal prolapse
- Perirectal abscess
- Anal fistula
- Infectious lesions

Presentation/Signs & Symptoms

- Anal mass
- Bleeding
- Itching
- Internal hemorrhoids are usually painless, unless thrombosis occurs
- External hemorrhoids are typically painful
- Sudden onset of excrutiating perirectal pain with palpable mass usually suggests acute thrombosis of a hemorrhoid

Diagnostic Evaluation

- Rectal exam
- Anoscopy
- Proctoscopy

Treatment/Management

- Treatment is initially conservative
    - High fiber diet
    - Appropriate anal hygiene
    - Sitz baths
    - Topical steroids
- Surgical options include rubber band ligation of internal hemorrhoids or surgical resection for large refractory hemorrhoids
- Acute thrombosis of a hemorrhoid may require drainage

Prognosis/Complications

- Only 4% of cases are symptomatic
- Most cases respond to medical treatment
- External hemorrhoids may result in thrombosis and eventual necrosis

Liver Disease

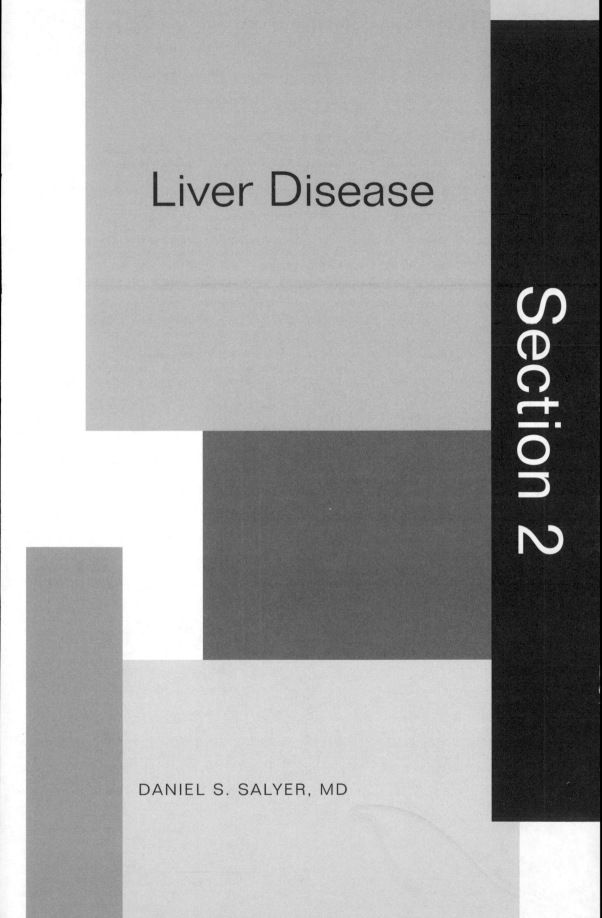

DANIEL S. SALYER, MD

Section 2

26. Liver Anatomy, Facts, and Pearls

- The liver is the largest parenchymal organ in the body
- Receives a dual blood supply via the portal venous system, which drains the gastrointestinal tract, and the hepatic arterial system via the aorta
- Hepatic blood flow is about 1500 mL/min, representing about 25% of cardiac output
  - 65–75% of hepatic blood flow arises from the portal vein
  - The hepatic artery contributes roughly half of the liver's oxygen supply
- Liver anatomy is divided into eight segments (I–VIII) based on portal venous blood supply
  - In the past, the liver was divided anatomically based on hepatic artery supply into a left and right lobe
  - The falciform ligament (the remnant of the umbilical vein) divides segments II and III from segment IV (medial and lateral segments of the left lobe)
  - The interlobar fissure is an imaginary line from the gallbladder fossa anteriorly to the inferior vena cava posteriorly that divides segments V and VIII from segment IV
- Venous drainage is via the hepatic veins to the inferior vena cava
- Variations in vasculature and biliary drainage are common and of surgical importance; for example, in 15–25% of the population, the left hepatic artery arises from the left gastric artery rather than the common hepatic artery
  - Due to the extreme variations in hepatic anatomy, surgeons often rely on pre-operative and intra-operative CT scans, ultrasound, MRA, and/or angiography to delineate the anatomy
- The triangle of Calot is an anatomic triangle bordered by the cystic duct, common hepatic duct, and the inferior border of the liver
  - In 75% of patients, the cystic artery is contained within the triangle of Calot
- The porta hepatis is composed of the common bile duct (anterolateral), common hepatic artery (anteromedial), and portal vein (posterior)
- Collateral connections between the portal and systemic circulations become important when portal hypertension results in backup of blood flow from the portal circulation to the systemic collateral channels
  - Esophageal varices results from dilatation of the connecting veins between the coronary vein and the azygous system
  - Caput medusae results from dilatation of the connecting veins between the umbilical vein in the falciform ligament and the epigastric veins in the abdominal wall
  - Hemorrhoids result from dilatation of the connecting veins between the superior hemorrhoidal vein and the middle and inferior hemorrhoidal veins
- The Pringle maneuver is a technique used by surgeons to temporarily compress the porta hepatis to reduce blood flow to the liver during surgery in order to control bleeding

27. Jaundice

Etiology/Pathophysiology

- Yellowish discoloration of skin, sclera, and mucous membranes, which occurs with an increase in concentration of serum bilirubin (jaundice becomes detectable when serum bilirubin exceeds 3 mg/dL)
- Pre-hepatic occurs due to increased production of bilirubin (unconjugated), which exceeds the liver's capacity to conjugate the extra load
  - Hemolytic disorders (e.g., hemoglobinopathies)
- Hepatic causes may be due to unconjugated hyperbilirubinemia or conjugated hyperbilirubinemia
  - Unconjugated cause is due to deficient (Gilbert's syndrome) or defective (Crigler-Najjar syndrome) glucuronyl transferase
  - Conjugated is due to hepatocellular injury (e.g., hepatitis, cirrhosis, tumors, toxins, drugs)
- Post-hepatic causes are due to obstruction of biliary drainage
  - Gallstones
  - Bile duct compression (e.g., pancreatitis, distal common bile duct tumor, pancreatic tumor)
  - Cholangitis, stricture, or bile duct tumor

Differential Dx

- Hemolysis
  - Hemoglobinopathies
  - Autoimmune
- Failure of bilirubin transport
  - Gilbert's syndrome
  - Crigler-Najjar syndrome
- Hepatocellular injury
  - Parenchymal liver injury (e.g., viral, toxins)
  - Hepatitis
  - Cirrhosis
- Cholestasis
  - Biliary obstruction
  - Choledocholithiasis
  - Carcinoma
  - Sclerosing cholangitis

Presentation/Signs & Symptoms

- Pre-hepatic jaundice is asymptomatic; patients may have a family history of splenectomy, anemia, or gallstones
- Patients with cirrhosis may present with ascites, edema, testicular atrophy, gynecomastia, encephalopathy, etc
- Cholestasis classically presents with jaundice, dark urine, pale stools, and pruritus
- Enlarged, tender liver suggests viral hepatitis
- Palpable, distended, painless gallbladder suggests carcinoma of the pancreas or distal bile duct (Courvoisier's sign)

Diagnostic Evaluation

- Initial tests include LFTs, urinalysis, and CBC
  - Elevated unconjugated bilirubin, anemia, elevated haptoglobin, and elevated reticulocyte count suggest hemolytic disease
  - Elevated conjugated and unconjugated bilirubin suggest cholestasis or hepatocellular injury
  - Elevated alkaline phosphatase suggests cholestasis
  - Elevated transaminases and LDH suggest hepatocellular injury
- Ultrasound is used to evaluate dilatation of the biliary tree, gallstones, and hepatic architecture
- ERCP or PTC are used to further evaluate ductal anatomy and allow for stenting of obstructed ducts and biopsy
- CT can identify obstructing mass lesions and evaluate hepatic parenchyma
- Biopsy is diagnostic for hepatocellular disease

Treatment/Management

- Treatment depends on the underlying cause
- Cessation of offending substances (e.g., alcohol, toxins, drugs)
- Surgical interventions may include:
  - ERCP with sphincterotomy or bile duct exploration to treat common bile duct stones and/or strictures, followed by cholecystectomy
  - Biliary tract decompression via ERCP with stenting, PTC, or choledochoenteric bypass
  - Resection of neoplasm (e.g., Whipple procedure)
  - Liver transplantation

Prognosis/Complications

28. Cirrhosis

Etiology/Pathophysiology

- Cirrhosis is the end result of prolonged hepatocellular injury, resulting in irreversible destruction, fibrosis, and nodular regeneration
- Most cases due to chronic alcohol abuse or viral hepatitis; however, any chronic liver disease (e.g., Wilson's disease, hemochromatosis, medications, primary sclerosing cholangitis, primary biliary cirrhosis) or massive acute injury (e.g., drug overdose) may result in cirrhosis
    - Most cases in the U.S. are due to chronic alcohol abuse and hepatitis C
    - Worldwide, the most common cause is schistosomiasis
- Clinical features result from hepatic cell dysfunction (e.g., decreased production of clotting factors and albumin), portal hypertension and porto-systemic shunting (e.g., esophageal varices, splenomegaly, caput medusae), and obstruction of bile flow (e.g., resulting in cholestasis, jaundice, elevated alkaline phosphatase)

Differential Dx

- First-degree biliary cirrhosis
- Second-degree biliary cirrhosis
- Noncirrhotic hepatic fibrosis (due to CHF and constrictive pericarditis)
- Budd-Chiari syndrome (hepatic vein thrombosis)
- Congenital hepatic fibrosis
- Partial nodular transformation
- Portal vein thrombosis (e.g., post-pancreatitis)
- α-1 antitrypsin deficiency

Presentation/Signs & Symptoms

- Patients often present with vague complaints of weight loss, fatigue, weakness, and malaise
- Anorexia, nausea, and vomiting
- Firm, nodular liver
- Signs of liver failure include jaundice, spider angiomas, palmer erythema, gynecomastia, testicular atrophy, bruising and hypocoagulation
- Signs of portal hypertension include ascites (abdominal distension, dyspnea), hepatosplenomegaly, caput medusae, and esophageal varices (GI bleeding)
- Hepatic encephalopathy: Lethargy, confusion, asterixis (flapping of hands when held out and flexed at the wrist), coma

Diagnostic Evaluation

- History is a key factor in diagnosis, with emphasis on alcohol use history, exposure to drugs and toxins, and history of viral infections
- LFTs are elevated early but decrease as liver is destroyed
    - AST and ALT reflect hepatocellular injury
- Alkaline phosphatase and GGTP reflect cholestasis
- Hypoalbuminemia, hypocholesterolemia, and decreased coagulation factors (increased PT/PTT/INR) imply defective hepatic hormone and protein synthesis
- Azotemia and electrolyte disturbances
- Abdominal ultrasound and CT scan provide evidence of abnormal liver architecture, ductal dilatation, hepatocellular carcinoma, and other abdominal pathology
- Percutaneous liver biopsy is diagnostic and may determine the underlying cause of cirrhosis
- Upper GI endoscopy will diagnose esophageal varices

Treatment/Management

- Treatment is aimed at preventing further hepatic deterioration and managing cirrhotic complications
- Hospitalize in acute deteriorations to manage complications (e.g., encephalopathy, GI bleeding)
- Avoid alcohol and potentially toxic medications
- Antiviral treatment for hepatitis B and C
- Administer lactulose to decrease protein absorption from the gut, thereby decreasing the production of ammonia and risk of azotemia and encephalopathy
- Manage ascites with dietary salt and protein restriction and diuretic therapy; if symptomatic, slowly remove ascitic fluid (rapid removal may result in hepatorenal syndrome)
- See "Portal Hypertension" entry for discussion of portosystemic shunting and variceal bleeding
- Liver transplantation

Prognosis/Complications

- Child's classification is used to assess hepatic functional reserve (includes three clinical variables and two biochemical variables)

Child's	A	B	C
Total Bilirubin	<2.0	2.0–3.0	>3.0
Albumin	>3.5	3.0–3.5	<3.0
Ascites	None	Controlled	Severe
Encephalopathy	None	Minimal	Coma
Nutrition	Good	Stable	Poor

- Mortality increases with higher Child's score
- Major complications include ascites, encephalopathy, bleeding esophageal varices, spontaneous bacterial peritonitis (infected ascitic fluid), hepatorenal syndrome, hepatocellular carcinoma, and death

29. Portal Hypertension

Etiology/Pathophysiology

- Increased resistance to blood flow through the portal vein, resulting in elevated portal venous pressure (>6 mmHg)
- Portal hypertension can be classified based on the location of the obstruction
  - Pre-hepatic causes: Narrowed portal vein, occlusive thrombosis
  - Intra-hepatic causes: Cirrhosis (most common cause in U.S.), schistosomiasis (most common cause worldwide), biliary cirrhosis, sarcoidosis, tuberculosis, and noncirrhotic hepatic fibrosis
  - Post-hepatic causes: Hepatic vein thrombosis (Budd-Chiari syndrome), inferior vena cava obstruction, right heart failure, constrictive pericarditis, restrictive cardiomyopathy

Differential Dx

- Portal hypertension secondary to extrahepatic causes
  - Adjacent inflammation (e.g., pancreatitis)
  - Obstructing mass
  - Splenic vein thrombosis
- Ascites secondary to extrahepatic causes
  - Nephrotic syndrome
  - Congestive heart failure
  - Carcinomatosis

Presentation/Signs & Symptoms

- GI bleeding secondary to esophageal varices
- Anorectal varices (hemorrhoids)
- Caput medusae
- Ascites
- Splenomegaly
- Hepatic encephalopathy
  - Mental status changes (e.g., confusion, stupor, coma)
  - Rigidity, hyperreflexia
  - Seizures
  - Asterixis (flapping of hands upon wrist flexion)
- Spontaneous bacterial peritonitis: Fever, abdominal pain, and tenderness
- Signs and symptoms of liver failure are outlined in the "Cirrhosis" entry

Diagnostic Evaluation

- Clinical presentation is often diagnostic
- Workup of liver failure and cirrhosis and its underlying etiology (see "Cirrhosis" entry)
- Upper GI endoscopy to document esophageal varices
- Abdominal ultrasound or CT scan to document ascites, liver architecture, and other abdominal pathology
- Measurement of portal vein pressure
  - Invasive measurements may be used; however, in practice, clinical findings are usually sufficient to diagnose elevated portal pressures
  - Portal vein pressure >6 mmHg is abnormal (esophageal varices begin to bleed at about 20 mmHg)
- Paracentesis and examination of ascitic fluid is indicated in patients with symptomatic ascites and signs of infection to rule out spontaneous bacterial peritonitis (SBP)
  - SBP is diagnosed by ascitic fluid with >1000 WBCs, >250 PMNs, or organisms

Treatment/Management

- Initial management of complications
- Treat bleeding esophageal varices by endoscopy with sclerotherapy, IV vasopressin or somatostatin, balloon tamponade, transjugular intrahepatic portosystemic shunt (TIPS), and surgical portosystemic shunting (see "Esophageal Varices" entry)
- Treat ascites by diuretics, sodium restriction, and therapeutic paracentesis
  - SBP requires IV antibiotics
- Treat hepatic encephalopathy by dietary protein restriction and lactulose (decreases protein absorption from the gut)
- Surgical reversal of portal hypertension may be accomplished by portosystemic shunting to bypass blood flow to the liver, including porto-caval shunt, mesocaval shunt, and distal splenorenal shunt
- Liver transplantation

Prognosis/Complications

- Esophageal varices can result in massive hematemesis and high mortality (>50%)
- Hepatorenal syndrome may result
- Child's classification is used to assess hepatic functional reserve

Child's	A	B	C
Total Bilirubin	<2.0	2.0–3.0	>3.0
Albumin	>3.5	3.0–3.5	<3.0
Ascites	None	Controlled	Severe
Encephalopathy	None	Minimal	Coma
Nutrition	Good	Stable	Poor

- Operative mortality of surgical shunting are directly related to Child's classification: Class A (0–5%), class B (10–15%), class C (>25%)
- Portosystemic shunt procedures may compromise the ability to later perform liver transplantation

30. Liver Abscess

Etiology/Pathophysiology

- Pyogenic (caused by bacteria) and amebic (caused by *Entamoeba histolytica*) liver abscesses are the most common types in the U.S.
  - Other types include parasitic, fungal, and mycobacterial
- Pyogenic abscess is often due to *Streptococci, Staphylococci, Klebsiella,* or *E. coli,* or *Bacteroides*
  - Most cases are secondary to direct spread from a biliary tract infection (e.g., ascending cholangitis)
  - Other causes include portal vein spread from GI infections (e.g., appendicitis, diverticulitis), systemic infection (e.g., endocarditis, bacteremia), and trauma (e.g., penetrating liver injury, recent ERCP or percutaneous transhepatic cholangiogram)
  - 60% of pyogenic abscesses occur in the right lobe, 20–25% bilateral, and <15% in the left lobe
  - Multiple abscesses occur in >30% of cases
- Amebic abscesses are common worldwide in tropical climates
  - Highest U.S. incidence occurs in the southern states
  - Caused by fecal-oral spread of *E. histolytica* cysts, which enter the liver via portal flow, lymphatics, or direct extension
- Parasitic (hydatid) abscess is often due to *Echinococcus granulosus*

Differential Dx

- Mass lesions (e.g., primary liver tumor)
- Hepatitis
- Cholangitis
- Cholecystitis
- Cystic liver disease
- Cholangiocarcinoma
- Other GI infections (e.g., gastroenteritis)
- Subphrenic abscess or other intra-abdominal abscess

Presentation/Signs & Symptoms

- Right upper quadrant pain is the most common presentation
- Pleuritic pain, right shoulder pain, or general pain may occur
- Signs of infection (e.g., fever, chills, night sweats)
- Jaundice
- Pruritus
- Enlarged, tender liver (often with a palpable mass)
- Often associated with diarrhea
- Sepsis may occur with pyogenic abscess
- Recent history of travel to endemic areas is suggestive of an amebic (e.g., South America, Mexico) or parasitic cyst (e.g., Mideast, Asia, Australia, Southern Europe)

Diagnostic Evaluation

- Laboratory abnormalities are generally non-specific and similar for all types of abscesses
  - Leukocytosis >15,000
  - Mild elevations of LFTs
  - Elevated bilirubin in some patients
- Right upper quadrant ultrasound is a useful first test and is best to identify amebic abscesses due to their large size
- Abdominal CT scan has better sensitivity than ultrasound
- A diagnosis of an amebic or parasitic abscess can be supported with serologic tests and stool examination
  - Anti-amebic serum antibody present in >95% of cases
- Needle aspiration and culture may be necessary if the diagnosis is in question
  - Amebic abscess will yield a sterile, odorless aspirate, often described as "anchovy paste"
  - Never aspirate a hydatid cyst due to the risk of fatal anaphylaxis upon leakage of cyst material

Treatment/Management

- The mainstay of therapy for pyogenic abscess is drainage and long-term antibiotics
  - Broad-spectrum antibiotics to cover aerobic and anaerobic organisms for 4–6 weeks
  - Drainage is generally accomplished percutaneously, with surgical exploration reserved for multiple abscesses or when percutaneous techniques fail
- Amebic abscess are treated with amebicidal drugs, principally metronidazole
  - Large or complicated abscesses (e.g., those blocking the bile duct or adjacent to the pericardium) may be aspirated
  - Surgical drainage is reserved for abscesses that have ruptured into the peritoneum
- Hydatid cysts are treated surgically by direct aspiration, irrigation, and removal of cyst wall

Prognosis/Complications

- Prognosis for properly treated pyogenic abscesses is often very good
  - Multiple abscesses and delayed diagnosis result in mortality of up to 40%
- Amebic abscess treated with amebicidals have a low mortality (about 1%)
  - Complications occur in 10–15% of patients, resulting in increased mortality
  - Complications include rupture into adjacent structures (e.g., pleura, pericardium, peritoneum)
- Hydatid cysts often rupture, resulting in formation of daughter cysts into adjacent viscera and/or anaphylactic shock
  - Anaphylactic shock due to parasitic cyst rupture is often fatal

31. Benign Liver Tumors

Etiology/Pathophysiology

- Hemangiomas are the most common benign tumor of the liver
  - Found in 8–10% the population
  - Divided into small capillary (most common) and cavernous hemangiomas (typically >4 cm)
  - Considered to be of congenital origin; however, a hormonal influence exists as females are affected more often than males and tumors are known to increase in size during pregnancy
- Focal nodular hyperplasia (FNH) is the second most common benign liver tumor
  - Found in 5–7% population
  - No clear link to oral contraceptive use
  - Females are affected much more often than males
  - Typically occurs in women of childbearing age
  - No risk of progression to hepatocellular carcinoma
- Hepatocelluar adenoma is much more common in women and strongly associated with oral contraceptive use
  - Risk is directly related to duration of exposure
  - Also associated with androgen use and some glycogen storage diseases
  - Increased risk of developing hepatocellular carcinoma

Differential Dx

- Malignant liver tumors
- Metastatic liver lesions
- Liver cyst
- Liver abscess
- Gallbladder cancer

Presentation/Signs & Symptoms

- Hemangiomas are generally asymptomatic and discovered incidentally
  - Large lesions can present with local mass effects (e.g., gastric outlet obstruction, jaundice) and pain
- Focal nodular hyperplasia is typically asymptomatic and found incidentally, but may produce vague abdominal complaints
- Hepatocelluar adenoma may result in symptoms due to mass effect
  - 30% of cases rupture and hemorrhage into the peritoneum, resulting in abdominal pain, hypotension, or shock

Diagnostic Evaluation

- Hemangiomas are diagnosed by MRI or CT with contrast
- Focal nodular hyperplasia is diagnosed by CT with contrast or ultrasound
  - A liver mass with a "central scar" on CT is highly suggestive of FNH (found in 30% of cases)
  - Technetium liver scan will show FNH but not an adenoma
- Hepatocelluar adenoma is typically diagnosed by CT or MRI
  - Biopsy may be necessary to exclude malignancy

Treatment/Management

- Hemangiomas, if asymptomatic, may be observed without specific treatment
  - Symptomatic lesions are treated with analgesics
  - Resection is only necessary for severe complications (e.g., hemorrhage) or persistent symptoms
- Focal nodular hyperplasia can be observed without specific treatment
  - Resection is indicated if symptomatic or if a malignant lesion cannot be ruled out
- Hepatocellular adenoma is generally resected due to the significant risk of rupture or hemorrhage, especially in the case of symptomatic or large lesions
  - Oral contraceptives or steroids should be discontinued
  - Pregnancy should be avoided due to risk of rupture

Prognosis/Complications

- Hemangiomas and focal nodular hyperplasia typically follow a benign course
- Hepatocellular adenoma that has ruptured and is bleeding has a very high mortality if surgical resection is attempted
  - Angiographic embolization should be performed immediately with later resection
  - If angiography is not immediately available, hepatic artery ligation is performed with later resection

32. Malignant Liver Tumors

Etiology/Pathophysiology

- By far, the most common liver malignancy is a metastatic tumor
  - The liver is the most common site for hematogenously spread metastatic disease (followed by the lung)
  - 12% of patients diagnosed with colorectal cancer will have isolated liver metastases
- The most common primary liver tumor is hepatocellular carcinoma (HCC); also known as hepatoma
  - Many diseases that result in chronic liver disease and cirrhosis predispose to hepatocellular carcinoma, including hepatitis B or C (75% of cases worldwide), alcoholic liver disease, hemochromatosis, Wilson's disease, schistosomiasis, and toxins (e.g., Aspergillus toxin, androgenic steroids, vinyl chloride, and thorotrast contrast)
- Cholangiocarcinoma is the second most frequent primary liver malignancy
  - Risk factors include primary sclerosing cholangitis and parasite infections
  - Klatskin tumor is a cholangiocarcinoma located at junction of the right and left hepatic ducts and results in total biliary obstruction
- Other primary malignant tumors include hepatoblastoma, sarcoma, and lymphoma

Differential Dx

- Benign liver tumors
- Liver cyst
- Liver abscess
- Cholecystitis
- Cirrhosis
- Budd-Chiari syndrome

Presentation/Signs & Symptoms

- Metastatic liver tumors are often asymptomatic and found on metastatic workup
- The classic presentation of HCC is right upper quadrant or epigastric pain (due to distention of liver capsule by the tumor and/or hemorrhage), abdominal swelling, and weight loss in a patient with existing cirrhosis
- Rarely, patients may present with jaundice due to compression of a large bile duct
- Paraneoplastic syndromes may occur, resulting in Cushing's syndrome, hypocalcemia, hypoglycemia, or hypertrophic pulmonary osteoarthropathy

Diagnostic Evaluation

- Serum α-fetoprotein and alkaline phosphatase are elevated in the majority of patients with hepatocellular carcinoma
- Ultrasound, CT scan, and MRI
- Angiography or MRA may be used to determine unresectability based on major vessel involvement
- Percutaneous liver biopsy is diagnostic; however, significant risk exists in the presence of cirrhosis and ascites; tumor seeding of the needle tract has been reported
- PET scanning may have a role in investigating liver tumors; currently under investigation

Treatment/Management

- Surgical management consists of complete resection of the lesion; however, most cases are unresectable at presentation
- Liver tumors derive the majority of their blood supply from the hepatic artery, which offers a treatment route for chemical embolization or placement of a continuous hepatic artery chemotherapy infusion pump
- Other modalities for the treatment of both metastatic disease and HCC include radiofrequency ablation, cryosurgery, and percutaneous ethanol injection
- Liver transplantation for HCC may offer some benefit in patients with cirrhosis and small, unresectable tumors

Prognosis/Complications

- Survival is generally very poor—death may occur in as little as 6–8 weeks from diagnosis
- Spread initially to remainder of liver and IVC
- Surgical resection can increase survival time 10-fold or more
- Liver transplant has resulted in 70–80% 5-year survival rates
- Recurrences of HCC range from 30–70% and are most often intrahepatic; original tumor size, number, grade, vascular invasion, and cirrhosis portend a higher recurrence rate
- 5-year survival after resection of colorectal metastases is estimated at 20–35%
- Prognosis of cholangiocarcinoma is poor

33. Liver Transplantation

Etiology/Pathophysiology

- Diseases potentially treated with liver transplantation include cirrhosis, primary sclerosing cholangitis, biliary atresia, hepatitis B and C, hemochromatosis, Wilson's disease, Niemann-Pick disease, glycogen storage diseases, Crigler-Najjar syndrome, α-1 antitrypsin deficiency, Budd-Chiari syndrome, fulminant hepatic failure, and selected patients with primary and metastatic cancers
- The most common indication for liver transplantation in adults is cirrhosis due to chronic alcohol abuse and hepatitis C
- The most common indication for liver transplantation in children is biliary atresia
- Some neoplastic processes can be treated with transplantation; typically slow growing tumors and those with low rates of recurrence (e.g., hepatoblastoma in children, hemangioendothelioma in adults)
    - Most other cancers are not candidates except some endocrine tumors and highly selected patients with hepatocellular carcinoma

Differential Dx

Presentation/Signs & Symptoms

- Presentations that may indicate the need for liver transplantation include increasing jaundice, severe pruritus, recurrent variceal bleeds, refractory ascites, refractory anti-coagulation, and worsening encephalopathy

Diagnostic Evaluation

- Candidates for transplantation are those with progressive, irreversible liver disease; no cancer or active infection; adequate renal, cardiac, and pulmonary reserve; no active substance abuse (alcoholics must have demonstrated abstinence); and age <65
- Candidates for cadaveric liver donor are those without history of liver disease or IV drug abuse; negative serologies for HIV and syphilis; no history of cancer (except some skin cancers or primary brain cancers); no abdominal or severe systemic infections; no significant hypoxia or hypotension; good cardiac, renal, and pulmonary function on support
- General laboratory values for acceptable donors include total bilirubin level <4.0 mg/dL, AST and ALT less than four times normal, alkaline phosphatase less than twice normal, and PT/PTT less than twice normal

Treatment/Management

- Orthotopic transplant: The donor liver is transplanted into the normal anatomic location following hepatectomy
- Heterotopic transplant: The donor liver is transplanted into a site other than the normal anatomic location
- Living transplant: A lobe or segment is obtained from a living donor
- Cadaveric transplant: Donor liver is transplanted from a deceased or brain dead person
- Split liver transplant: A cadaveric donor liver is divided to be used in two recipients

Prognosis/Complications

- Survival after transplantation is generally good
    - 85% 1-year survival for adults
    - 60% 10-year survival
- Complications of transplantation include post-operative intra-abdominal bleeding, hepatic artery or portal vein thrombosis, bile duct leak or obstruction, and infections due to immunosuppresion
- Transplantation recipients with hepatitis C often see a recurrence within a year post-transplantation, which often mimics rejection

Gallbladder Disease

Section 3

JOHN J. RAVES, MD
SCOTT KAHAN, MD
JASON W. COTTER, MD

34. Gallbladder Anatomy, Facts, and Pearls

Gallbladder Anatomy

- The fundus is the anterior tip of the gallbladder
- The body is the main bile storage area
- The infundibulum is the most posterior portion of the gallbladder, located between the neck and the body
- The neck connects the body to the cystic duct
- The cystic duct connects the gallbladder to the bile duct

- The gallbladder is a gastrointestinal organ that stores bile
- The functions of the gallbladder are storage of bile, concentration of bile via absorption of water and electrolytes, release of bile upon stimulation from the vagus nerve and cholecystokinin
- Located in the right upper quadrant of the abdomen beneath the inferior aspect of the right lobe of the liver
- The triangle of Calot is an anatomic triangle bordered by the cystic duct, common hepatic duct, and the inferior border of the liver
  - In 75% of patients, the cystic artery is contained within the triangle of Calot
- Blood supply is from the cystic artery, which usually arises from the right hepatic artery
- Bile from the gallbladder drains through the cystic duct, which joins the common hepatic duct to become the common bile duct
- Bile is composed of lipids (including cholesterol, lecithin, and bile salts), bile pigments, water, and electrolytes
- The anatomy and blood supply of the gallbladder and biliary tract can be quite variable and anomalous; "normal anatomy" occurs in only about 50% of patients; if anatomic variations are not recognized, major complications may occur during surgical procedures

35. Cholelithiasis/Biliary Colic

Etiology/Pathophysiology

- Gallstones (cholelithiasis) are found in at least 10% of the population
  - 80% of patients are asymptomatic and will not develop sequelae
  - Some cases may result in intermittent stone obstruction at the neck of the gallbladder, causing episodic pain (biliary colic)
  - May also result in chronic obstruction and progression to cholecystitis (infection and inflammation of the gallbladder) and/or cholangitis (infection and inflammation of the common bile duct, which may result in sepsis and shock)
  - Significant but "silent" gallbladder disease may occur in diabetics and immunosuppressed patients due to poor pain perception and impaired inflammatory responses; these patients often present late in the course of the disease, often with severe cholecystitis or sepsis
- Stones may be composed of cholesterol (75%), pigments, or mixed
- The classic risk factors for cholesterol stones are *female*, *forty*, *fat*, *fertile*
- Other risk factors include bile stasis, chronic hemolysis, oral contraceptives, rapid weight loss, obesity, total parenteral nutrition, and ileal resection
- Other causes of biliary colic include a non-functional or dysfunctional gallbladder (biliary dyskinesia) and cholesterolosis of gallbladder

Differential Dx

- Cholecystitis
- Peptic ulcer disease
- Hepatitis
- Liver abscess
- Gastritis
- Pancreatitis
- Carcinoma of the liver or bile ducts
- Carcinoma of the gallbladder
- Cholangitis
- Biliary obstruction
- Right lower lobe pulmonary disease (e.g., PE, pneumonia)
- Myocardial ischemia

Presentation/Signs & Symptoms

- Episodic RUQ/epigastric pain
  - Usually transient (<12 hours)
  - Colicky (comes and goes)
  - Often postprandial
  - Pain may radiate to back, right scapula, or right shoulder
- Food intolerance (especially fatty, greasy, or fried foods, meats, and cheeses)
- Dyspepsia, eructation (burping)
- Nausea/vomiting
- RUQ tenderness and/or a palpable gallbladder may be present

Diagnostic Evaluation

- History and physical examination
- CBC, liver function tests, amylase, and lipase
- Ultrasound will directly show gallstone shadows
  - Will also reveal evidence of cholecystitis, if present, such as wall thickening and pericholecystic fluid
- HIDA scan with CCK stimulation may diagnose biliary dyskinesia and may also be indicated to rule out cystic duct obstruction and acute cholecystitis
  - In cases of biliary dyskinesia, the gallbladder will not empty despite CCK stimulation
- Rule out choledocholithiasis (gallstones in the bile ducts), which will present with elevated bilirubin in a patient with a history of jaundice or cholangitis
- Chest X-ray and ECG are useful to rule out cardiopulmonary disease
- Abdominal X-rays will reveal gallstones in 10% of cases

Treatment/Management

- Avoid fatty foods and other triggers of biliary colic
- Cholecystectomy is the treatment of choice for symptomatic disease
  - Laparoscopic (preferable) or open
  - Intra-operative cholangiogram should be used if there is a history of elevated LFTs or amylase, suspicion of choledocholithiasis, or if the ductal anatomy is unclear
  - Lithotripsy may be used to break up stones in patients who are not surgical candidates
- Asymptomatic cholelithiasis need not be treated
  - Consider cholecystectomy in immunocompromised or diabetic patients who have asymptomatic stones due to possible "silent" disease

Prognosis/Complications

- The most common complication is obstruction of the gallbladder, resulting in cholecystitis, empyema, and/or hydrops of the gallbladder
- Choledocholithiasis and/or cholangitis occur less commonly
- Migration of stones to the intestines via a cholecystoenteric fistula may result in a gallstone ileus

36. Cholecystitis

Etiology/Pathophysiology

- Infection and inflammation of the gallbladder, thought to occur secondary to partial or complete obstruction of the cystic duct
- >95% of cases are associated with gallstones
- The remainder of cases are due to acalculous cholecystitis (gallbladder inflammation in the absence of stones), which usually occurs in high risk patients (e.g., post-surgical patients)
- Risk factors include patients who are *female, fertile, fat, forty, flatulent*
- Other risk factors include diabetes mellitus, steroid or oral contraceptive use, bile stasis, cirrhosis, hyperlipidemia, chronic hemolysis, and immunosuppresssion
- May result in abscess formation, cholangitis, sepsis, and/or shock

Differential Dx

- Peptic ulcer disease
- Hepatitis
- Liver abscess
- Gastritis
- Pancreatitis
- Carcinoma of the liver or bile ducts
- Carcinoma of the gallbladder
- Cholangitis
- Biliary obstruction
- Right lower lobe pulmonary disease (e.g., pulmonary embolism, pneumonia)
- Myocardial ischemia

Presentation/Signs & Symptoms

- RUQ pain/tenderness
- Fever
- Nausea/vomiting
- Right subscapular pain
- Right shoulder pain (referred from irritation of diaphragm)
- Gallbladder is palpable and painful in one-third of cases
- Murphy's sign: Palpation of the RUQ during inspiration results in inspiratory arrest secondary to pain

Diagnostic Evaluation

- Appropriate history and physical is highly suggestive of gallbladder disease
- CBC will reveal leukocytosis
- Elevations of LFTs, amylase, bilirubin, and alkaline phosphatase may represent choledocholithiasis (stones in the common bile duct)—immediate decompression of the biliary tree is necessary via ERCP, percutaneous transhepatic cholangiogram (PTC), or open common bile duct exploration
- Ultrasound is the gold standard for diagnosis of gallbladder pathology: May show distended gallbladder, thickened walls, pericholecystic fluid, and stones
- Hepatobiliary nuclear scan (HIDA scan) may be used if the diagnosis is in doubt; evaluates for cystic duct obstruction and/or acute cholecystitis
- CT may be used but it is somewhat less accurate and much more expensive than ultrasound

Treatment/Management

- Administer IV fluids and broad-spectrum antibiotics
  - Common infectious agents include enteric gram-negative rods (*E. coli* and *Klebsiella*), *Enterococcus*, and anaerobes (e.g., *Bacteroides*)
  - Ampicillin or first generation cephalosporin will cover most gram negatives and *Enterococcus*
  - Metronidazole may be added to cover anaerobes
- Nasogastric decompression if patient is vomiting
- Cholecystectomy is the treatment of choice
  - Laparoscopic cholecystectomy if possible
  - Open cholecystectomy
  - Percutaneous cholecystostomy may be used to decompress the gallbladder in high risk patients who cannot tolerate surgery
- Sphincterotomy via ERCP in patients with choledocholithiasis may be curative or preventive

Prognosis/Complications

- Very good prognosis if treated early
- Complications include abscess formation, perforation, and formation of a cholecystoenteric fistula with subsequent gallstone ileus
- Complications of cholecystectomy include wound infection, bleeding or hematoma formation, subphrenic or subhepatic abscess, and bile leak (cystic duct leak or injury to common bile duct)
- Though many people have asymptomatic cholelithiasis, few cases will result in cholecystitis—however, once infection occurs, surgery to remove the gallbladder is indicated as cholecystitis is likely to recur

37. Cholangitis

Etiology/Pathophysiology

- Inflammation and bacterial infection of an obstructed common bile duct, which may progress to sepsis and shock
  - *E. coli* is the most common causative organism
- Most commonly caused by gallstones in the common duct
- Other causes include post-operative strictures of the bile duct, obstructive neoplasms, sclerosing cholangitis, plugged biliary drainage tubes (e.g., T tube), or during injection of contrast solution into the biliary tree (e.g., ERCP, PTC, or intra-operative cholangiography)

Differential Dx

- Cholecystitis
- Peptic ulcer disease
- Hepatitis
- Liver abscess
- Gastritis
- Pancreatitis
- Carcinoma of the liver or bile ducts
- Carcinoma of the gallbladder
- Biliary obstruction

Presentation/Signs & Symptoms

- RUQ/epigastric pain
- Pain may radiate to back, right scapula, or right shoulder
- Nausea/vomiting
- Charcot's triad is present in the majority of cases: Fever, jaundice, and RUQ pain
- Reynold's pentad: Fever, jaundice, RUQ pain, shock, and mental status changes
- Peritoneal signs may be present
- Patients may present with sepsis or septic shock

Diagnostic Evaluation

- History and physical examination with presence of Charcot's triad is strongly suggestive of cholangitis
- CBC will reveal leukocytosis
- Elevated LFTs (especially bilirubin and alkaline phosphatase) suggest obstructive jaundice
- Ultrasound may reveal common bile and hepatic duct dilatation

Treatment/Management

- Resuscitate patients with IV fluids and pressors as needed
- Administer broad-spectrum IV antibiotics to cover gram negatives and anaerobes (e.g., first generation cephalosporin and metronidazole)
- Treatment is aimed at relieving the biliary duct obstruction
  - ERCP with papillotomy if stones are the etiology
  - Surgery (e.g., common duct exploration, biliary-enteric bypass) may be necessary to treat strictures or retained stones
  - Biliary drainage via PTC catheter
  - Unplugging of blocked biliary drain

Prognosis/Complications

- Cholangitis generally resolves following decompression
- Overall prognosis depends on the cause of the obstruction
  - Stones and strictures usually have a good outcome following treatment
  - Malignancies and sclerosing cholangitis have poor long-term outcomes

38. Choledocholithiasis

Etiology/Pathophysiology

- Stones in the bile ducts
  - Gallstones originate in the gallbladder and are passed into the common bile duct and/or hepatic ducts
  - In rare instances, primary bile duct stones may form in a patient who has had a prior cholecystectomy
- 4% of patients with cholelithiasis are found to have choledocholithiasis, without symptoms of common bile duct obstruction

Differential Dx

- Cholecystitis
- Peptic ulcer disease
- Hepatitis
- Liver abscess
- Gastritis
- Pancreatitis
- Carcinoma of the liver or bile ducts
- Carcinoma of the gallbladder
- Cholangitis
- Biliary obstruction
- Right lower lobe pulmonary disease (e.g., PE, pneumonia)
- Myocardial ischemia

Presentation/Signs & Symptoms

- Episodic RUQ/epigastric pain
- Nausea/vomiting
- Intermittent jaundice
- Dark urine (bilirubinuria)
- Acholic stools
- Gallbladder is most often non-palpable as opposed to a malignant obstruction of the bile ducts (e.g., pancreatic cancer, distal bile duct cancer, ampullary cancer)
- May be asymptomatic

Diagnostic Evaluation

- Elevated LFTs (especially bilirubin and alkaline phosphatase) suggest obstructive jaundice
- Ultrasound may reveal common bile and hepatic duct dilatation; rarely, a common bile duct stone may be identified
- Endoscopic retrograde cholangiopancreatography (ERCP) is diagnostic to visualize stone in the bile ducts
- Percutaneous transhepatic cholangiography (PTC) may also be used to visualize the ducts; however, this is a more invasive test than ERCP
- HIDA scan may show biliary duct obstruction but is less useful than other diagnostic tests in the presence of elevated bilirubin

Treatment/Management

- Treatment is directed at removing the obstructing bile duct stone and removing the gallbladder and its stones to prevent further stone migration into the biliary tree
- Laparoscopic cholecystectomy with common bile duct exploration and extraction of stone(s) may be attempted; however, conversion to an open procedure is often necessary
- ERCP with basket stone retrieval and papillotomy may alternatively be done
  - ERCP is successful at clearing the ducts in 90% of cases
  - Elective cholecystectomy (laparoscopic or open) should follow ERCP decompression

Prognosis/Complications

- There is a 5–10% incidence of retained stones following surgical or ERCP stone removal
- Retained stones may be treated by chemical dissolution or biliary-enteric bypass (e.g., choledochoduodenostomy, choledochojejunostomy)
- Complications of ERCP include pancreatitis and perforation of the duodenum

39. Gallbladder Cancer

Etiology/Pathophysiology

- Rare (4% of all cancers)
- Present in 1% of patients who undergo biliary tract surgery
- 90% of patients have cholelithiasis
- 4 times more common in females
- There is a strong association (up to 50%) between the presence of a porcelain gallbladder (calcified gallbladder wall) and gallbladder carcinoma

Differential Dx

- Cholecystitis
- Peptic ulcer disease
- Hepatitis
- Liver abscess
- Gastritis
- Pancreatitis
- Carcinoma of the liver or bile ducts
- Cholangitis
- Biliary obstruction
- Right lower lobe pulmonary disease (i.e., PE, pneumonia)
- Myocardial ischemia

Presentation/Signs & Symptoms

- The majority of cases present with symptoms of cholecystitis
  - RUQ pain/tenderness
  - Fever
  - Weight loss
  - Nausea/vomiting
  - Right subscapular pain
  - Right shoulder pain (referred from irritation of diaphragm)
  - Painful and/or palpable gallbladder
  - Murphy's sign: Palpation of the RUQ during inspiration results in inspiratory arrest secondary to pain
- Obstructive jaundice may be a late presentation

Diagnostic Evaluation

- The majority of cases are discovered during planned cholecystectomy
- Ultrasound and abdominal CT may reveal stones and a mass in or around the gallbladder
- Abdominal X-ray may reveal the presence of a porcelain (calcified) gallbladder
- Liver function tests may be elevated in late stages secondary to obstructive jaundice

Treatment/Management

- Cholecystectomy is curable only if the carcinoma is discovered incidentally and is confined to the gallbladder
- Unfortunately, most cases already invade the liver and gallbladder fossa at the time of surgery; wedge resection of liver may be attempted but is rarely curative

Prognosis/Complications

- Prognosis is extremely poor: 5-year survival of <10%
- Complications include lymphatic or hepatic metastases, obstruction, bleeding, or fistula

Pancreatic Disease

Section 4

JASON W. COTTER, MD

40. Pancreas Anatomy, Facts, and Pearls

- The pancreas in an endocrine and exocrine gland located in the retroperitoneum
- Composed of a head, neck, uncinate, body, and tail
- Anterior to the first and second lumbar vertebrae, the aorta, and the portal vein
- Posterior to stomach
- Intricately involved with the superior mesenteric artery and vein
- Tail of the pancreas is directly adjacent to the spleen and contains the splenic artery
- The ductal system consists of the main duct of Wirsung, which enters the duodenum (along with the common bile duct) at the ampulla of Vater, and an accessory duct of Santorini, which enters the duodenum at the minor papilla
- Pancreatic divisum: Congenital failure of fusion of the pancreatic ducts results in the minor duct (Santorini) acting as the main draining duct
- Annular pancreas: Congenital abnormality of pancreatic development resulting in pancreatic tissue that completely surrounds the duodenum and may cause duodenal obstruction

41. Acute Pancreatitis

Etiology/Pathophysiology

- Inflammation of pancreas due to inappropriate activation of pancreatic enzymes within and surrounding the pancreas, resulting in autodigestion, necrosis, edema, and possibly hemorrhage
- Disease varies from a mild, self-limited course to severe pancreatitis with hemorrhagic necrosis leading to systemic multi-organ failure and death
- 80% of acute attacks are due to alcohol or cholelithiasis
  - The usual cause of gallstone pancreatitis is a gallstone passing out of the gallbladder into the bile duct; the stone either passing through or obstructing the distal bile duct incites the pancreatitis
- Less common etiologies include hyperlipidemia, hypercalcemia, drugs (e.g., thiazide diuretics, steroids), infections (e.g., mumps), scorpion bites, trauma, iatrogenic (e.g., ERCP), and idiopathic

Differential Dx

- Peptic ulcer disease
- Gastritis
- Cholecystitis
- Cholangitis
- Hepatitis
- Liver abscess
- Ruptured abdominal aortic aneurysm
- Mesenteric ischemia
- Appendicitis
- Diverticulitis
- Renal colic
- Lower lobe pulmonary disease
- Myocardial ischemia

Presentation/Signs & Symptoms

- Steady, severe epigastric pain
  - Generally begins 1–4 hours after large meal or alcohol intake
  - Radiation to back
  - Relieved by leaning forward
- Nausea/vomiting
- Abdominal distension
- Severe cases may present with signs of peritonitis (e.g., guarding, rebound tenderness, fever), dehydration, and profound shock
- Hemorrhagic pancreatitis may present with ecchymoses or bluish discoloration of the umbilicus (Cullen's sign) or flank (Turner's sign)

Diagnostic Evaluation

- Initial laboratory studies include CBC, liver function tests, amylase, and lipase
  - Lipase and amylase are generally elevated in acute disease (lipase has higher specificity than amylase since amylase is also found in other tissues)
  - The degree of amylase/lipase elevation does *not* correlate with severity of the pancreatitis
  - Electrolyte abnormalities include hypokalemia and hypocalcemia
  - Elevated LFTs and LDH in biliary disease
- Plain films are non-specific and may show dilated sentinel bowel loop, left pleural effusion, atelectasis, and will rule out pneumonia and perforation
- Abdominal CT is insensitive for pancreatitis but may reveal phlegmon (inflammatory mass), pseudocyst, or abscess
- Ultrasound has poor sensitivity for pancreatic pathology but will show associated biliary tract disease (e.g., stones)

Treatment/Management

- Supportive care is the mainstay of treatment
  - Aggressive IV fluid replacement (normal saline) is necessary due to third spacing into retroperitoneal space—titrate fluids to maintain urine output
  - Bowel rest (NG tube, NPO) in severe disease
  - Administer meperidine for pain (morphine may cause sphincter of Oddi dysfunction)
  - Antiemetics as necessary
  - Monitor and correct electrolyte abnormalities (especially calcium)
- Determine and treat the specific etiology (e.g., avoid alcohol, undergo cholecystectomy once pancreatitis resolves)
- Indications for surgery include biliary or pancreatic duct obstruction, severe pancreatitis that doesn't respond to treatment, abscess/necrosis requiring drainage, and pseudocyst formation

Prognosis/Complications

- Ranson's criteria are used to assess severity and determine prognosis

On admission	After 48 hours
• Age >55	• HCT decrease by >10%
• WBC >16	• BUN increase >5
• Glucose >200	• Ca^{++} <8
• LDH >350	• PaO_2 <60
• AST >250	• Base deficit >4
	• Fluid resuscitation >6 L

- For each positive criteria, there is approximately 10% increased associated mortality
- >90% mortality if six or more criteria are present
- Complications include splenic vein thrombosis, abscess or pseudocyst formation, necrosis, ARDS, sepsis, and multiple organ system failure

42. Chronic Pancreatitis

Etiology/Pathophysiology

- Chronic pancreatitis is a slowly progressive destruction of pancreatic tissue from inflammation, fibrosis, and distortion of the pancreatic ducts
- Most commonly due to alcohol abuse
- Other causes include cystic fibrosis, severe protein calorie malnutrition, hyperparathyroidism, obstruction of pancreatic duct, and idiopathic

Differential Dx

- Pancreatic cancer
- Other GI malignancy
- Biliary colic
- Cholecystitis
- Gastritis
- Peptic ulcer disease
- Abdominal aneurysm
- Mesenteric ischemia
- Intestinal obstruction
- Lower lobe pulmonary disease
- Myocardial ischemia

Presentation/Signs & Symptoms

- Chronic epigastric pain, often radiating to the back
- Nausea/vomiting
- Food intolerance and/or signs of malnutrition
- Steatorrhea
- Jaundice
- Glucose intolerance

Diagnostic Evaluation

- Classic triad of pancreatic calcifications, steatorrhea, and diabetes (impaired glucose intolerance)
- In contrast to acute pancreatitis, amylase and lipase are usually not elevated and leukocytosis often absent
- Abdominal CT scan may show pancreatic calcifications, chronic inflammation, or atrophy
- Abdominal X-rays show pancreatic calcifications in some cases
- Endoscopic retrograde cholangiopancreatography (ERCP) or magnetic resonance cholangiopancreatography (MRCP) are the gold standards for diagnosis
- Rule out pancreatic cancer with CEA, CA 19-9, and biopsy if necessary

Treatment/Management

- Avoid alcohol and fatty foods
- Replace pancreatic enzymes and vitamins B_{12}, A, D, E, K
- Administer meperidine for pain
- Administer insulin or hypoglycemic agents if diabetes is present
- Surgical intervention may include resection (pancreatectomy) or drainage of dilated pancreatic ducts (Puestow or Duval procedures)
  - Puestow procedure: Side-to-side pancreaticojejunostomy
  - Duval procedure: Distal pancreatectomy with pancreatic-jejunal anastomosis
- Pancreatic pseudocysts may be surgically drained by forming an anastomosis between the pseudocyst and the stomach or the jejunum (after waiting 4–6 weeks for the pseudocyst wall to mature)

Prognosis/Complications

- Poor prognosis if alcohol is the cause and patient continues to drink—50% mortality at 10 years
- Prognosis is good if patient remains abstinent and replacement therapy is adequate
- Patients have increased risk of pancreatic cancer
- Pancreatic pseudocyst formation (non-epithelialized collection of pancreatic fluid)
  - Small cysts may resolve without intervention
  - Large cysts may be complicated by bleeding, infection, or obstruction
- Narcotic addiction

43. Pancreatic Cancer

Etiology/Pathophysiology

- Fourth most common cause of cancer
- Etiology is unclear
  - Tobacco use is probably the greatest risk factor
  - May also be associated with caffeine and alcohol use, diabetes, and asbestos exposure
- 70% occur in head of pancreas, 20% in body, 10% in tail
- Usually age >50

Differential Dx

- Chronic pancreatitis
- Peptic ulcer disease
- Other GI malignancies
- Biliary obstruction
- Hepatitis
- Gastritis

Presentation/Signs & Symptoms

- Insidious onset of weight loss, fatigue, anorexia, and gnawing abdominal or back pain
- Epigastric pain with radiation to the back is probably the most common symptom but *painless jaundice* is a common presentation
- Pain may improve with bending forward
- Jaundice, dark urine, acholic stools
- Pruritus
- Palpable, non-tender gallbladder (Courvoisier's sign)
- Migratory thrombophlebitis

Diagnostic Evaluation

- Initial laboratory analysis includes CBC, LFTs, amylase, and lipase
  - Alkaline phosphatase and bilirubin elevated if bile duct is obstructed or if liver metastases present
- Tumor associated antigens (CEA and CA 19-9) may be elevated
- Abdominal CT should be the first test
- Ultrasound, endoscopic ultrasound (most accurate for staging), and ERCP may enhance the sensitivity of CT and are useful for staging
- MRI, MR with angiography (MRA), or laparoscopy may be used to determine resectability
- Percutaneous or open biopsy for definitive diagnosis

Treatment/Management

- Resection is the only truly effective treatment
- Pancreaticoduodenectomy (Whipple's procedure) is performed to remove cancerous tissue while preserving GI continuity
  - Removal of the duodenum, head of the pancreas, and gallbladder with re-anastomosis of the common bile duct to the jejunum (choledochojejunostomy), pancreas to the jejunum (pancreaticojejunostomy), and stomach to the jejunum (gastrojejunostomy)
- Total or distal pancreatectomy may be performed
- If the tumor is unresectable, palliation of bile duct and GI tract obstructions may be accomplished by choledochojejunostomy, gastrostomy, and jejunostomy
- Radiation and chemotherapy for palliation
- Liberal use of narcotics for pain control in unresectable disease

Prognosis/Complications

- Nearly all patients have advanced tumors and local or widespread metastases at the time of diagnosis
  - Patients with back pain at initial presentation nearly always have unresectable disease due to local extension to the retroperitoneum
- Very poor prognosis (5-year survival <5%)
- Median survival in patients with unresectable cancer is <6 months
- Curative operations are only possible in 10–15% of patients—usually only for tumors in the head of the pancreas, which cause early jaundice but have not yet spread to lymph nodes
- Complications of surgery include abscess and anastomotic leaks

44. Insulinoma

Etiology/Pathophysiology

- A pancreatic β cell tumor that releases abnormally large amounts of insulin
- 10% are malignant

Differential Dx

- Exogenous insulin administration
- Pheochromocytoma
- Carcinoid
- Syncope secondary to neurologic or cardiac etiologies
- Multiple endocrine neoplasia

Presentation/Signs & Symptoms

- Palpitations
- Nervousness
- Mental status changes
- Signs and symptoms of hypoglycemia (e.g., syncope)
- Whipple's triad
  - Hypoglycemia
  - Illness precipitated by fasting
  - Illness relieved with glucose intake
- Adenopathy may be present in malignant metastatic tumors

Diagnostic Evaluation

- Increased insulin in the presence of low glucose levels is pathognomonic for insulinoma
- Proinsulin level will differentiate insulinoma from exogenous administration of insulin (>20% of total circulating insulin in cases of insulinoma)
- Rule out MEN type I by checking serum calcium to rule out hyperparathyroidism
- CT scan, MRI, and/or angiogram may be necessary to localize the tumor

Treatment/Management

- Surgical excision is the cornerstone of treatment
- Enucleation or distal pancreatectomy may be done if there is no suspicion of malignancy
- If firm lymph nodes are felt, formal cancer surgery, such as a pancreaticoduodenectomy, should be performed
- Intra-operative ultrasound may be necessary to help localize the tumor
- In cases where the tumor cannot be localized, consider total pancreatectomy versus pancreaticoduodenectomy

Prognosis/Complications

- 65% of cases are cured with surgery
- Malignant insulinoma carries a 60% 2-year survival
- Intra-operative monitoring for hypoglycemia

Vascular Disease

CHRISTOPHER G. JOHNNIDES, MD

45. Vascular Anatomy, Facts, and Pearls

Carotid Artery
- Lies in the carotid sheath along with the internal jugular vein and vagus nerve
- Ascends in the neck medial to the internal jugular vein
- The common carotid artery has no branches and bifurcates into the external and internal carotid arteries at the level of the superior rim of the thyroid cartilage; the facial vein often marks the level of the bifurcation
- The external carotid artery has several branches and supplies structures of the neck, larynx, and face
- The internal carotid artery supplies the brain
- The hypoglossal nerve, vagus nerve, and glossopharyngeal nerve are at risk of injury during carotid endarterectomy; the ansa cervicalis and the superior laryngeal nerve also can be injured

Aorta
- The great vessels of the thoracic aorta include the inominate artery (which gives rise to the right subclavian and common carotid arteries), the left common carotid artery, and the left subclavian artery
- Blood supply to the spinal cord comes from intercostals that arise from the thoracic aorta; the artery of Adamkiewicz is important in providing blood supply to the spinal cord and may be injured following thoracic aortic surgery
- The abdominal aorta has the following important branches: Renal, celiac, superior mesenteric, and inferior mesenteric arteries
- The mesenteric circulation consists of the three main branches of the abdominal aorta: Celiac trunk supplies stomach and duodenum; superior mesenteric artery supplies jejunum, ileum, and right colon; inferior mesenteric artery supplies left colon and rectum
- The meandering mesenteric artery, or the arc of Riolan, is a continuous arterial link between the left branch of the middle colic (from the SMA) and the left colic (from the IMA) arteries; it often becomes enlarged in cases of mesenteric occlusive disease
- The aorta bifurcates into the common iliac arteries, which each bifurcate into the external and internal iliac (or hypogastric) arteries

Lower Extremities
- The external iliac artery continues into the groin as the common femoral artery; this divides into the superficial and deep femoral (profundus) arteries
- As the superficial femoral artery exits the adductor canal (Hunter's canal) just above the knee, it becomes the popliteal artery; this artery has components that extend above and below the knee
- Below the knee, the popliteal artery gives rise to the "trifurcation": This describes the branching of the anterior tibial artery (laterally) and the tibioperoneal trunk, which divides into the tibial and peroneal arteries
- The term "run-off" is used to describe the angiographic appearance of these three vessels as they approach the ankle

- In all cases of vascular surgery for atherosclerotic disease, the leading cause of death is myocardial infarction

46. Abdominal Aortic Aneurysm

Etiology/Pathophysiology

- Dilatation of the aorta >3 cm due to weakening of the aortic wall from loss of elastin and collagen
- Atherosclerosis, hypertension, connective tissue diseases (e.g., Takayasu's arteritis), Marfan syndrome, age >60, male sex, family history, tobacco use, peripheral vascular disease, and vasculitis predispose to the development of AAA
- The abdominal aorta is the most common site of aortic aneurysms; >90% originate below the renal arteries
- Once present, aneurysms typically grow 0.3–0.5 cm/year
- Untreated AAA may result in rupture of the aneurysm, a catastrophic event with high mortality
    - Patients with a ruptured AAA have a 30–50% chance of dying before reaching the hospital
    - Patients that undergo emergent surgical repair have mortality of 40–50%
    - Elective repair reduces mortality to <5%
- Bacteria account for 5% of AAAs (*Staphylococcus, Salmonella*, syphilis)
- Embolization of thrombi formed within the aneurysm may result in ischemia of viscera or lower extremities

Differential Dx

- Aortic dissection
- Pancreatitis
- Peptic ulcer disease/GERD
- Diverticulitis
- Mesenteric ischemia
- Cholecystitis/biliary colic
- Renal colic
- Musculoskeletal pain
- Other causes of syncope (e.g., aortic stenosis, cardiac arrhythmia)
- Myocardial ischemia
- Acute pulmonary disease (e.g., pneumonia, pneumonitis)

Presentation/Signs & Symptoms

- AAA is usually asymptomatic
    - Vague abdominal or back pain, abdominal bruit or pulsatile abdominal mass may be present
    - Palpation of aneurysm may be difficult, especially in obese patients
    - Early satiety, nausea, or vomiting may occur due to duodenal compression
- Ruptured or leaking aneurysms may present with severe back, abdominal, or flank pain that may radiate to the groin
    - Hypotension and tachycardia
    - Syncope
    - Abdominal mass on exam
    - Signs of retroperitoneal hematoma (Grey-Turner's or Cullen's signs)

Diagnostic Evaluation

- History and physical examination
    - Palpation of an aneurysm may be difficult, depending on body habitus and obesity
- CT scan, MRI, or ultrasound may all be used for diagnosis and to monitor progression of aneurysm size
    - Ultrasound is the most cost effective method to monitor size
    - CT scan is most accurate (e.g., for surgical landmarks)
- Angiography is rarely indicated unless renal hypertension, iliofemoral occlusive disease, horsehoe kidney, or mesenteric ischemia is suspected
    - Angiogram reveals only the internal lumen of the vessel but not the entire aneurysm sac
- Clinical suspicion of a ruptured or leaking AAA with a bedside ultrasound in the ED that identifies an aneurysm is sufficient to proceed to the operating room

Treatment/Management

- Asymptomatic AAAs discovered incidentally require only outpatient vascular surgery follow-up
    - If <4.5 cm, follow with serial ultrasounds, avoid tobacco, lower blood pressure and lipids
    - If >4.5 cm, elective surgery indicated due to risk of rupture
- Indications for surgery
    - Symptomatic and/or ruptured or leaking aneurysms
    - Size >4.5 cm
    - Rapidly enlarging aneurysms (>0.5 cm/year)
    - Evidence of embolization to lower extremities from aneurysm thrombus
- Current surgical technique
    - Open repair with prosthetic graft
    - Endovascular repair (percutaneous placement of intraluminal stents) carries a lower operative mortality rate

Prognosis/Complications

- Normal enlargement rate is 0.4 cm/year
- Rupture risk correlates with size
    - 4.0–5.4 cm: 0–1.0% risk of rupture per year
    - 6.0–7.0 cm: 6.6% risk of rupture per year
    - >7 cm: 19% risk of rupture per year
- 50% peri-operative mortality following rupture
- <5% elective peri-operative mortality
- Postoperative complications include cardiac ischemia, hemorrhage, graft infection, aortoenteric fistula, ureteral injuries, renal failure, ileus, colonic ischemia, distal embolization, paraplegia, and impaired sexual function
    - GI bleeding in any patient with an abdominal aortic graft is considered to be due to an aortoenteric fistula until proven otherwise
    - The most common cause of death after an aneurysm repair is an MI
- Ultrasound screening of family members

47. Thoracic Aortic Aneurysm

Etiology/Pathophysiology

- Thoracic aortic aneurysms may involve the ascending, transverse, or descending thoracic aorta
- Predisposing factors include atherosclerosis, tobacco use, hypertension, and COPD
- Aneurysms of the aortic arch are usually secondary to atherosclerosis and Marfan syndrome
  - In the past, syphilitic aortitis was a common cause
- Aneurysms of the descending thoracic aorta are usually secondary to atherosclerosis or trauma
- Thoraco-abdominal aneurysms extend across the diaphragm to involve the upper abdominal aorta and are usually secondary to atherosclerosis
  - Often involves the origins of the celiac, superior mesenteric, and renal arteries
- Crawford classification for thoracic aneurysms
  - I: Involves the descending aorta up to (but not below) the renal arteries
  - II: Involves all or most of the descending thoracic and abdominal aorta
  - III: Distal descending aorta and some of the abdominal aorta
  - IV: All or most of the abdominal aorta, including the suprarenal portion involving the visceral vessels

Differential Dx

- Aortic dissection
- Abdominal aortic aneurysm
- Pancreatitis
- Peptic ulcer disease
- Hiatal hernia
- Musculoskeletal pain
- Myocardial ischemia
- Mediastinal mass (e.g., lymphoma, lung cancer, esophageal cancer, thymoma)

Presentation/Signs & Symptoms

- Pain (chest, back, flank, or abdominal) is the most common symptom
- Hoarseness secondary to stretching of the recurrent laryngeal nerve
- Dyspnea or other pulmonary symptoms may occur due to bronchial or lung compression
- Proximal thoracic aneurysms may result in symptoms of aortic regurgitation
- Superior vena cava syndrome may occur
- Asymptomatic aneurysms commonly present as an abnormal chest X-ray revealing a mediastinal mass

Diagnostic Evaluation

- Chest X-ray may reveal a mediastinal mass or retrocardiac shadow
- CT scan and MRI (or MRA) will delineate the size and extent of the aneurysm and will determine surgical landmarks
- Transesophageal echocardiography may also reveal the aneurysm and evaluate for aortic regurgitation
- Angiography may be helpful in thoraco-abdominal aneurysms to determine involvement of the mesenteric and renal arteries

Treatment/Management

- Open vascular repair with insertion of graft
- Endovascular stenting may soon replace current open surgical procedures
- Cardiopulmonary bypass or temporary aortic shunting techniques are often necessary during open repair

Prognosis/Complications

- 60% 5-year survival after repair
- Complications of surgery include spinal ischemia, paraplegia, hemorrhage, renal failure, bowel ischemia, and complications of atherosclerosis (e.g., MI, CVA)

48. Aortic Dissection

Etiology/Pathophysiology

- Underlying cystic medial necrosis of the thoracic aorta results in a tear of the intima, separating the layers of the aortic wall
- Predisposing factors include hypertension, atherosclerosis, tobacco use, Marfan syndrome, male gender, pregnancy (third trimester), tertiary syphilis, trauma, and coarctation of the aorta
- 80–90% of patients are older than 60
- Dissection may also involve the abdominal aorta (may result in renal and/or mesenteric artery occlusion) or coronary arteries (may cause MI)
- DeBakey classification
  - I: Dissection involves the ascending aorta and extends beyond aortic arch
  - II: Involves the ascending aorta only
  - IIIa: Involves the descending aorta, but is contained above the diaphragm
  - IIIb: Involves the descending aorta and descends below the diaphragm
- Stanford classification
  - A: Dissection of ascending aorta (may or may not involve the transverse or descending aorta)
  - B: Dissection of the descending aorta only
- Aortic dissection has been erroneously referred to as a "dissecting aneurysm"—it is not an aneurysm or aneurysmal disease

Differential Dx

- Myocardial infarction
- GERD
- Esophageal spasm
- Acute pericarditis
- Pulmonary embolus
- Pneumothorax
- Cholecystitis
- Peptic ulcer disease
- Extremity arterial occlusion
- Cerebrovascular accident

Presentation/Signs & Symptoms

- Acute onset of severe, tearing chest pain that radiates to the back
- Associated with nausea, diaphoresis, dyspnea, tachycardia, neurologic symptoms (e.g., syncope, paresthesias)
- Hypertension
- Proximal dissection: Diminished upper limb pulses and blood pressure; possible coronary involvement (heart block, aortic regurgitation, CHF, MI)
  - Hypotension may occur if proximal dissection results in hemopericardium and tamponade
- Distal dissection: Diminished lower limb pulses and blood pressure, oliguria, mesenteric ischemia

Diagnostic Evaluation

- Chest X-ray is 90% sensitive for dissection
  - Widened mediastinum
  - Blurred aortic knob
  - Deviation of the trachea to the right
  - Elevation of the right mainstem bronchus and depression of the left bronchus
  - Pleural effusion
  - Cardiomegaly (pericardial effusion)
- ECG may show non-specific changes (e.g., LVH, ischemia) and is used to rule out MI
- Transesophageal echocardiogram (TEE) is the imaging test of choice
- Chest CT or MRI may also be used in stable patients
- Angiography was previously the gold standard, but is now used less frequently as its sensitivity is only 80%; also used for surgical landmarking

Treatment/Management

- Medical therapy is aimed at decreasing blood pressure and diminishing myocardial contractility (e.g., β-blockers, nitrates)
- Surgical intervention depends on the type of dissection
  - Emergent surgery for proximal dissections (Stanford A or DeBakey I/II)
  - Distal dissections (Stanford B or DeBakey III) usually requires only medical therapy; however, surgical repair is warranted in cases of aortic rupture, limb ischemia, and renal or gut ischemia
  - Endovascular stenting may soon replace current open surgical procedures
- Acute decompensation requires supportive therapy, including bed rest, β-blockers to keep SBP <120, IV fluids if hypotensive secondary to tamponade, and surgery as necessary

Prognosis/Complications

- Ascending dissections have a much worse prognosis
  - Mortality increases by 1% per hour during the first 48 hours
  - 60% mortality in the first month without surgical intervention
  - <10% peri-operative mortality for elective repairs
- Distal dissections have <10% mortality after 1 month without surgical intervention
- Postoperative complications (5–10%) include paraplegia, MI, renal insufficiency, mesenteric ischemia, and impotence

49. Peripheral Vascular Disease

Etiology/Pathophysiology

- Atherosclerotic obstructive disease of the arteries of the lower extremities (and, less often, of the upper extremities)
- Risk factors include hyperlipidemia, diabetes mellitus, smoking, and hypertension
- Affects 5% of 50–70 year old patients and 10% of people >70 (approximately 10 million people in the U.S.)
- Limb-threatening ischemia occurs when arterial blood flow is insufficient to meet the metabolic needs of resting tissue
- Diabetic peripheral vascular disease accounts for >60% of leg amputations in the U.S.

Differential Dx

- Lumbar spinal stenosis: "Pseudoclaudication" (usually bilateral pain and paresthesias in the lower extremities upon walking or standing—symptoms abate with sitting or bending forward)
- Thromboangiitis obliterans (Buerger disease)
- Popliteal artery entrapment
- Deep venous thrombosis
- Radicular back pain

Presentation/Signs & Symptoms

- Intermittent claudication is the characteristic symptom
    - Lower extremity discomfort with exercise (pain, tightness, cramping)
    - May be unilateral or bilateral
    - Presents at a relatively constant walking distance
    - Symptoms disappear upon resting
    - In severe arterial obstruction, symptoms may continue even at rest
- Decreased or absent peripheral pulses
- Arterial bruits
- Pallor of feet upon exercise or elevation
- Muscle atrophy, hair loss, thickened toenails, skin fissures, shiny skin
- Severe disease results in ulceration, tissue necrosis, and gangrene

Diagnostic Evaluation

- History and physical exam—diagnosis is usually made clinically
- Fontaine classification:
    - Stage I: Asymptomatic
    - Stage II: Intermittent claudication
    - Stage III: Rest and nocturnal pain
    - Stage IV: Necrosis, gangrene
- Non-invasive testing may include ankle:brachial index <1 and/or significant drop with exercise, segmental leg pressures, duplex ultrasound, or magnetic resonance angiography
    - Ankle:brachial index and segmental pressures may be inaccurate in diabetic patients with severe calcific atherosclerosis
- Peripheral angiography is a highly accurate, though invasive method of testing; used only if surgical intervention is planned

Treatment/Management

- Medical treatment includes lifestyle modification (e.g, smoking cessation, diabetes control, blood pressure lowering, exercise) and various drug therapies (low dose aspirin, clopidogrel, pentoxifylline, cilostazol)
- Endovascular techniques may include angioplasty and stent placement
- Surgical revascularization (bypass) is indicated for ischemia, peripheral emboli, impotence, and in patients with lifestyle-limiting symptoms
    - Pre-operative evaluation is mandatory (e.g., cardiac and cerebral risk factors)
    - Bypass is accomplished by autologous saphenous vein grafts or synthetic grafts (e.g., Gore-tex, Dacron)
    - Vein grafts have better patency rates compared to synthetic materials

Prognosis/Complications

- Peripheral vascular disease is a marker of atherosclerotic disease—affected patients have a high incidence of coronary artery and cerebrovascular disease
    - 5- and 10-year mortality rates are directly related to coronary and cerebral disease
- 75% of patients with claudication improve with conservative therapy
- Complications include acute arterial occlusion, hemorrhage, graft or wound infection, pseudo-aneurysm formation, and gangrene requiring amputation
- Operative mortality is 1–3%, with most deaths due to cardiac events

50. Carotid Artery Occlusive Disease

Etiology/Pathophysiology

- Approximately 500,000 people per year suffer from strokes, leading to 200,000 deaths per year (third most common cause of death in the U.S.)
- Carotid artery disease is the most common cause of stroke in the U.S.
- A *transient ischemic attack* (TIA) is a temporary ischemic event that resolves completely within 24 hours
- A *stroke in evolution* is an acute neurologic event that progresses to a major cerebral infarct within hours to days
- Cerebrovascular accident (stroke) may occur due to disruption of blood flow of the anterior cerebral circulation (carotid system) or the posterior cerebral circulation (vertebrobasilar system)
- Carotid artery occlusive disease is due to atherosclerosis
    - Atherosclerotic lesions commonly occur at the carotid bifurcation (due to high flow differentials, high shear stress, and turbulent flow), resulting in reduced blood flow to the cranial circulation
    - Ultimately, cerebral disease most commonly occurs due to embolization from the carotid plaque (emboli may consist of clot, platelet aggregates, or cholesterol)

Differential Dx

- Vertebrobasilar cerebral disease
- Emboli of cardiac origin (e.g., arrhythmia, valvular disease, endocarditis)
- Non-atherosclerotic carotid lesions (e.g., Takayasu's arteritis, fibromuscular dysplasia, radiation injuries)
- Intracranial hemorrhage
- Hematologic disorders (e.g., sickle cell disease)
- Intracerebral neoplasm
- Hypoglycemia
- Epilepsy
- Migraine
- Psychogenic

Presentation/Signs & Symptoms

- May be asymptomatic
- Focal neurologic deficits on the contralateral side
    - Motor deficits or paralysis (e.g., inability to move arm)
    - Paresthesias
    - Weakness
- Language deficits (expressive or cognitive aphasia)
- Amaurosis fugax is a reliable sign of a carotid TIA
    - Described as a curtain coming down over the patient's eye
    - Caused by occlusion of a branch of the ophthalmic artery
- A carotid bruit may or may not be present

Diagnostic Evaluation

- Carotid duplex ultrasound is the primary screening modality to evaluate for carotid artery stenosis or occlusion
- Cerebral angiography or magnetic resonance angiography provide further detail and greater accuracy of the degree of the stenosis; however, may dislodge clots and precipitate an embolic stroke
- CT scan or MRI of the brain may be indicated to evaluate for infarcts, hemorrhage, and other cerebral pathology
- Further diagnostic tests may include cardiac workup (e.g., ECG, echocardiogram, TEE), CBC, glucose, chemistries, ESR, serum lipids, uric acid, thyroid function tests, and hypercoagulable workup

Treatment/Management

- Anticoagulation (e.g., coumadin) and antiplatelet therapy (aspirin, clopidogrel) reduce the risk of stroke in patients with prior stroke or TIA
- Carotid artery endartectomy is the removal of offending atherosclerotic plaque in the common, internal, and/or external carotid arteries
    - Proven indications for surgery include symptomatic patients with high grade carotid stenosis (>70%) or asymptomatic patients with stenosis >70%, or recurrent TIAs despite medical therapy
- Emergent administration of heparin and/or antithrombolytic agents may be indicated in acute embolic events

Prognosis/Complications

- Recurrent stroke is the leading cause of death in stroke patients
- Recurrent stroke rates
    - In symptomatic patients with stenosis ≥70%, 26% of patients treated with medical management alone will have a further stroke within 2 years versus 9% of patients treated with surgery
    - In asymptomatic patients with stenosis ≥70%, 11% of patients treated with medical management alone will have a further stroke within 5 years versus 5% of patients treated with surgery
- Postoperative complications include stroke (<3%), myocardial infarction, cranial nerve palsies, and wound complications (e.g., bleeding, infections)

51. Mesenteric Ischemia

Etiology/Pathophysiology

- There are four primary etiologies: Embolization, thrombosis of pre-existing atherosclerotic lesion, nonocclusive mesenteric ischemia, and mesenteric venous thrombosis
- Acute mesenteric ischemia occurs due to sudden occlusion of a previously normal mesenteric artery or thrombosis of the mesenteric veins
  - Arterial occlusion is most commonly embolic secondary to a proximal source (e.g., atrial fibrillation, cardiac thrombus, atherosclerotic or aneurysmal disease of the proximal aorta)
  - Emboli may also be secondary to thrombus formation in a mesenteric artery beyond a proximal stenotic occlusion
  - Venous thrombosis most commonly occurs due to hypercoagulable states (e.g., myeloproliferative disorder) or low blood flow states (e.g., heart failure)
- Chronic mesenteric ischemia (intestinal angina) occurs when at least two mesenteric arteries are narrowed or occluded secondary to chronic atherosclerotic disease
- Ischemic colitis is a non-occlusive (never embolic) process involving the IMA that occurs secondary to low flow states (e.g., CHF, hypercoagulable states)

Differential Dx

- Perforated viscus (e.g., duodenal/gastric ulcer)
- Intestinal obstruction
- Abdominal aortic aneurysm
- Aortic dissection
- Pancreatitis
- Cholelithiasis
- Inflammatory bowel disease
- Hernia
- Volvulus
- Intussusception
- Diverticulitis
- Colon cancer
- Infectious colitis

Presentation/Signs & Symptoms

- Acute mesenteric ischemia: Sudden onset of severe abdominal pain, often out of proportion to physical exam
  - Vomiting, diarrhea, and occult blood may be present
  - Physical exam may be unremarkable
  - Hypoactive or absent bowel sounds
  - Peritonitis (guarding, rigidity, rebound tenderness) and hypotension occur late
- Chronic mesenteric ischemia is characterized by crampy, dull *postprandial* abdominal pain
  - Abdominal bruit may be present
  - Weight loss (patients may avoid eating)
- Ischemic colitis: Episodes of crampy LLQ pain, hematochezia, and diarrhea

Diagnostic Evaluation

- If peritonitis or shock are present, proceed directly to OR
- Acute mesenteric ischemia
  - Leukocytosis; metabolic acidosis; and elevated LDH, CPK, alkaline phosphatase, and lactate may be present
  - Abdominal X-ray may reveal dilated loops of bowel
  - Late changes on CT (after bowel infarction and necrosis occurs) include edema, bowel wall thickening, pneumotosis intestinalis
  - Angiography is the gold standard for arterial occlusion and may be therapeutic by infusion of vasodilators or thrombolytics
  - Mesenteric venous thrombosis can be diagnosed by CT
- Chronic mesenteric ischemia
  - Angiography is diagnostic
  - Duplex ultrasound
- Ischemic colitis is diagnosed by barium enema (thumbprinting) or colonoscopy (edema, ischemic mucosa)

Treatment/Management

- Volume resuscitation, antibiotics, and anticoagulation
- Acute mesenteric ischemia
  - If signs of perforation are present (e.g., peritonitis), exploratory laparotomy is necessary
  - Angiography with administration of thrombolytics, vasodilators, or angioplasty with stent placement
  - Surgical intervention with goal of revascularization if possible and resection of non-viable bowel
  - A planned "second look" 24–36 hours after the initial surgery to assess viability of the remaining bowel
- Mesenteric venous thrombosis is treated by thrombolysis, long-term anticoagulation, and possible resection of non-viable bowel
- Chronic mesenteric ischemia: Surgical revascularization via percutaneous transluminal angioplasty, endarterectomy, or vascular bypass
- Ischemic colitis: Supportive care with antibiotics, bowel rest, and hydration; surgery is rarely needed

Prognosis/Complications

- A high index of suspicion is necessary as mortality is directly related to delay of diagnosis and treatment
- Acute mesenteric ischemia: 50% 5-year survival
- Chronic mesenteric ischemia, 70% 5-year survival
- Patients are at increased risk of sepsis due to mucosal breakdown and invasion
- Complications of surgery include bleeding, intestinal leak, further intestinal ischemia, stricture formation, and MI

52. Renovascular Hypertension

Etiology/Pathophysiology

- Renovascular hypertension due to renal artery stenosis is thought to account for up to 5% of cases of hypertension
- Renal artery stenosis occurs secondary to atherosclerosis or fibromuscular dysplasia; activation of renin-angiotensin-aldosterone axis results in systemic vasoconstriction (due to angiotensin II) and volume expansion (due to aldosterone)
- Atherosclerotic lesions predominantly affect the renal ostium, whereas fibromuscular dysplasia affects the long segments of the renal artery and its branches
- When there is a significant lesion of one renal artery but a normal contralateral kidney, the contralateral kidney will compensate for the activated renin-angiotensin-aldosterone system; however, when both renal arteries are stenotic, no compensation is possible
- 30% of patients with multivessel coronary disease have evidence of renal artery stenosis; however, not all patients will have hypertension
- Hypertension that is not responsive to medical therapy is suggestive of a secondary cause (e.g., renal artery stenosis, chronic kidney disease, pheochromocytoma, Cushing's disease)

Differential Dx

- Essential hypertension
- Chronic kidney disease
- Pheochromocytoma
- Hyperaldosteronism
- Coarctation of the aorta
- Hyperthyroidism
- Drugs (e.g., cocaine, amphetamines, oral contraceptives, alcohol, steroids, sympathomimetics)

Presentation/Signs & Symptoms

- Severe hypertension with a negative family history, sudden elevation of BP, and/or onset before age 20 or after 50
- Signs and symptoms of end-organ damage may be present (e.g., retinal hemorrhage, heart failure)
- Flank bruit may suggest fibromuscular dysplasia (young women > men)
- Localized epigastric bruit may suggest atherosclerotic renal artery stenosis
- Hypertension is often severe and refractory to medications

Diagnostic Evaluation

- The basic workup for hypertension is a complete history and physical, urinalysis, BUN/creatinine, chemistries, and assessment of cardiac target organ damage via ECG and/or echocardiogram
- Focused studies are reserved for patients with the above clinical features or who have severe or refractory HTN
- Renal angiography provides definitive diagnosis
- MRA and captopril renal scintigraphy may be used
- Renal duplex ultrasound is operator-dependent but may be helpful for diagnosis
- Renal vein assays (renal vein sampling for renin) can assess for an ischemic kidney (increased renin) and a compensating kidney (suppressed renin)

Treatment/Management

- Medical management of hypertension
- Endovascular techniques (balloon angioplasty with or without stenting) may be used
- Surgical management may include aortorenal bypass, endarterectomy, extra-anatomic bypass (e.g., hepatorenal or splenorenal bypass), ex vivo reconstruction, or nephrectomy

Prognosis/Complications

- Endovascular treatment for fibromuscular dysplasia of the main renal artery is effective in 50% of patients
- Endovascular treatment for atherosclerotic lesions is less effective, with a 30% restenosis rate after 1 year
- Operative mortality is about 3%, primarily due to cardiovascular events
- Surgical intervention for atherosclerotic disease provides a cure for 15% of patients but controls hypertension in 75% of patients
- Surgical intervention for fibromuscular dysplasia provides a cure in 45% of patients
- In patients with ischemic nephropathy, a properly timed operation can halt decline in renal function and prevent progression to dialysis

53. Venous Insufficiency

Etiology/Pathophysiology

- The venous system of the lower extremities is composed of superficial veins (outside the deep fascia and muscles) and deep veins (within the muscular compartments)
  - Venous insufficiency is a disorder of the deep veins
  - Varicose veins are a disorder of the superficial veins
  - Incompetence of perforating veins, which connect the deep and superficial veins, allows high venous pressures to be transmitted from the deep compartments to the superficial system, resulting in varicose veins
- The etiology of venous insufficiency and varicosities is poorly understood; genetics, hormones (progesterone and estrogen), and environment (acquired valve damage, prolonged standing) have all been implicated
- The primary disorder of venous insufficiency and varicose veins is incompetence of the venous valves
- Half of adult working men and two-thirds of adult working women have varicose veins; up to 20% of the working population has severe chronic venous insufficiency
- Primarily a disease of western civilization

Differential Dx

- Arterial insufficiency
- Deep venous thrombosis
- Cellulitis
- Systemic causes of pedal edema (e.g., CHF, nephrotic syndrome, liver failure)

Presentation/Signs & Symptoms

- Extremity swelling
- Pruritus
- Easy tiring and feelings of fatigue
- Symptoms may be relieved with recumbency or leg elevation
- Skin pigmentation and induration occurs as venous insufficiency progresses
- Malleolar ulcers develop in severe cases

Diagnostic Evaluation

- History and physical examination
- Doppler venous ultrasound can accurately map the veins in the leg and identify valvular and perforator incompetence
- Computer-assisted air displacement plethysmography allows measurement of venous filling
- Venography is rarely used

Treatment/Management

- Medical therapy includes bed rest, graduated compressive stockings, and antibiotics for phlebitis
- Venous ablation with injection of sclerosing agent into the vein
- Vein stripping/ligation
- Open or endoscopic subfascial ligation of the incompetent perforating vein
- Direct venous reconstruction (veno-veno bypass and autogenous valve transplant) for deep venous insufficiency if medical therapy fails

Prognosis/Complications

- Direct sclerosis or ligations of superficial varicose veins has a high success rate
- Perforator interruption combined with superficial ablation has a 75–85% success rate at controlling venous ulceration
- Complications of venous insufficiency and varicose veins include hemorrhage, phlebitis, and skin ulceration
- Complications of surgery include hemorrhage, wound infection, and recurrence or worsening of varicosities

Breast Disease

Section 6

MARY BETH MALAY, MD

54. Breast Anatomy, Facts, and Pearls

- The breast is a tear-shaped gland that lies ventral to the pectoralis major muscle
- Functional elements of the breast include the alveoli (where milk is produced), which are grouped into lobules, and the ducts, which serve as a conduit to the nipple
- Cooper's ligaments are bands of connective tissue within the breast that act as supporting structures
- Arterial supply is via the internal mammary artery and lateral thoracic artery (from axillary artery)
- Venous drainage is via the axillary vein, internal mammary veins, and intercostal veins
- Axillary lymphatics account for 97% of lymphatic drainage

Three Levels of Axillary Drainage:
- Level 1 is lateral to or below the pectoralis minor
- Level 2 is deep to and behind the pectoralis minor
- Level 3 is medial to or above the upper border of the pectoralis minor
- Minor lymphatic drainage from the internal mammary chain (3%)
- Rotter's nodes are interpectoral lymphatic tissue between the pectoralis major and minor muscles

Nerves of Surgical Significance:
- The long thoracic nerve (nerve of Bell) provides motor function to the serratus anterior muscle; damage results in a winged scapula
- The thoracodorsal nerve provides motor function to the latissimus dorsi muscle; damage may result in mild shoulder weakness
- The intercostal brachial nerve provides sensation to the skin of the medial aspect of the upper arm; damage results in numbness
- The lateral pectoral nerve innervates the pectoralis major muscle; damage may lead to atrophy of the pectoralis muscle

55. Benign Breast Disease

Etiology/Pathophysiology

- Benign lesions may be characterized according to their risk for malignant transformation
  - Low risk lesions include fibrocystic changes, cysts, and fibroadenomas
  - Moderate risk lesions include atypical ductal hyperplasia and atypical lobular hyperplasia
  - High risk lesions include lobular carcinoma in situ (LCIS), which is a marker for the potential development of breast cancer (usually an incidental discovery during pathologic examination of a breast tissue sample)
- Breast tissue is very sensitive to the cyclic hormonal variations of the menstrual cycle
  - Some benign lesions, namely fibrocystic changes and cysts, commonly exhibit cyclic variations with menses
  - Malignant lesions rarely fluctuate in size with the menstrual cycle

Differential Dx

- Breast carcinoma
- Cystosarcoma phyllodes
- Fat necrosis
- Hematoma
- Breast abscess
- Intramammary lymph node

Presentation/Signs & Symptoms

- Breast pain and/or tenderness
- Breast "lumpiness"
- Palpable mass

Diagnostic Evaluation

- Obtain risk factors to determine the risk for malignancy (e.g., personal or family history of breast cancer, early menarche, late menopause, nulliparity, older age at first full-term delivery, hormone replacement therapy)
- Physical exam, including breast examination with careful attention to area(s) of palpable mass
- Bilateral mammogram should be the initial test; however, may not be helpful if <age 35 due to high breast density
- Ultrasound is used in conjunction with mammography to further delineate lesions
  - Used for masses that cannot be seen on mammogram
  - Used to determine whether a palpable mass and/or a lesion identified on mammogram is solid or cystic
- Fine needle aspiration of solid masses or symptomatic cysts for cytology will distinguish benign from malignant cells
- Core needle biopsy of solid lesions and/or complex cysts provides a definitive tissue diagnosis

Treatment/Management

- Fibrocystic changes, simple cysts, and fibroadenomas do not mandate surgical removal; however, cysts and fibroadenomas warrant close follow-up with monthly self-breast exams and 6-month physical exams, mammogram, and/or ultrasound
- Recurrent cysts following aspiration, large (>3 cm) fibroadenomas, or enlarging fibroadenomas should be excised
- Atypical ductal or lobular hyperplasia requires either close surveillance with a mammogram and breast exam every 6 months or surgical excision of the area
- LCIS requires close follow-up with clinical exam and mammography
  - Patients with LCIS who are at very high risk for breast cancer may decide to undergo bilateral mastectomy

Prognosis/Complications

- Malignant transformation of benign breast conditions can occur
  - Low risk lesions (1.5–2 times increased risk) include fibrocystic changes, cysts, and fibroadenomas
  - Moderate risk lesions (4–5 times increased risk) include atypical ductal hyperplasia and atypical lobular hyperplasia
  - High risk lesions (8–10 times increased risk) include lobular carcinoma in situ (LCIS)

56. Malignant Breast Disease

Etiology/Pathophysiology

- 1 in 8 lifetime risk of developing breast cancer in U.S. women
- Incidence of breast cancer increases with age, but slows after menopause
- At the time of diagnosis, 90% of patients will have localized disease
- Increased levels of circulating estrogens are associated with an increased development of breast cancer (e.g., hormone replacement therapy, uninterrupted menstrual cycles—nulliparity, early menarche, late menopause)
- Risk factors include hereditary breast cancer syndromes (e.g., mutations in BRCA-1 and BRCA-2 genes, which result in a 50–85% lifetime risk of developing breast cancer), personal history of breast cancer, family history of breast cancer, early menarche, late menopause, nulliparity, atypical ductal hyperplasia, and long-term hormone replacement therapy
- Premalignancies: Ductal (intraductal) carcinoma in situ (DCIS), lobular (intralobular) carcinoma in situ (LCIS)
- Invasive carcinomas: Infiltrating ductal carcinoma, infiltrating lobular carcinoma, medullary carcinoma
- Inflammatory carcinoma: A poorly differentiated, highly aggressive cancer that may be of ductal or lobular origin (see associated entry)
- Paget's disease of the breast: Tumor cells invade nipple and areola

Differential Dx

- Benign breast disease
  - Fibrocystic changes
  - Cysts
  - Fibroadenoma
  - Atypical hyperplasia (ductal or lobular)
  - Intraductal papilloma
- Breast abscess
- Fat necrosis
- Hematoma

Presentation/Signs & Symptoms

- Abnormal mammogram may be the only presentation
- Breast lump
- Skin thickening/erythema
- Peau d'orange (localized edema of the dermal lymphatics, resulting in gross visibility of the overlying skin pores) may occur in advanced tumors that approach the dermis
- Nipple inversion/crusting may occur with tumors underneath the nipple or areola or in cases of Paget's disease
- Bloody nipple discharge
  - Intraductal papilloma is the most common cause of bloody discharge
  - Ductal carcinoma must be considered in older patients
- Enlarged axillary/supraclavicular lymph nodes

Diagnostic Evaluation

- History (e.g., risk factors) and physical exam
- Bilateral mammogram is the initial test; however, may not be helpful if <age 35 due to high density of breast tissue
- Ultrasound is used as an adjunct to mammography to delineate masses that cannot be seen on mammogram and to determine whether a lesion is solid or cystic
- Biopsy of palpable lesions
  - Fine needle aspiration extracts cells for cytologic examination to distinguish benign versus malignant lesions
  - Core needle biopsy of solid lesions or complex cysts is used to extract tissue and provide a definitive diagnosis
  - Excisional biopsy (lumpectomy) is definitive and may be curative if the full lesion is removed
- Biopsy of non-palpable lesions or suspicious calcifications on mammogram may be evaluated by core needle biopsy (either ultrasound-guided or stereotactic) or removed by needle localized surgical excision
- MRI/PET scans may be considered for indeterminate mammogram and/or ultrasound results

Treatment/Management

- Preferred treatment is breast conservation surgery (lumpectomy followed by radiation therapy) or mastectomy—no survival difference between lumpectomy plus radiation versus mastectomy
- Combination chemotherapy is given to most patients with invasive cancer regardless of nodal status; may be given pre-operatively (neoadjuvant) to downsize large tumors to permit breast conservation surgery
- Hormone therapy is used for estrogen and/or progesterone receptor-positive patients
  - Administer tamoxifen for 5 years to improve disease-free survival, decrease local tumor recurrence, and decrease the risk of contralateral breast cancer
  - Tamoxifen is contraindicated in patients with a history of thromboembolic events
  - Aromatase inhibitors may be an alternative to tamoxifen in postmenopausal females, which may reduce the risk of thromboembolism formation

Prognosis/Complications

- Metastatic workup must be done
- 5-year survival rate of all patients with breast cancer is 85%
- Pathologic exam of lesions are required to determine nodal status (the most predictive indicator overall), tumor size, histology, and hormone receptor status
  - Positive axillary nodes portend the worst prognosis
  - Larger tumors (>5 cm) have a poorer overall survival
  - Poorly differentiated and higher grade tumors have a worse outcome
  - Presence of estrogen or progesterone receptors carries a better prognosis
  - Presence of HER-2/neu receptor may be a marker of more aggressive disease

57. Inflammatory Breast Disease

Etiology/Pathophysiology

- Inflammatory carcinoma is a poorly differentiated, highly aggressive cancer, which may be of ductal or lobular origin
- The most aggressive form of breast carcinoma
- Constitutes 1–4% of all breast cancers
- A clinical and pathologic entity defined by dermal lymphatic invasion of the breast by tumor cells
- Nodal involvement and distant metastases are common at initial presentation
- Often mistaken for a breast infection or abscess because it presents with erythema, warmth, and induration
    - Many patients are initially treated with antibiotics, resulting in a delay of diagnosis
    - A high index of suspicion is necessary if a suspected breast infection does not rapidly improve with antibiotic administration

Differential Dx

- Breast infection/abscess
- Advanced breast cancer

Presentation/Signs & Symptoms

- Increased size and firmness of the breast
- Diffuse brawny induration of the breast with erythema and edema
- Breast may be warm to the touch
- An underlying breast mass may or may not be present
- Nipple retraction may occur
- Palpable axillary and/or supraclavicular nodes may be present
- May have associated arm edema secondary to lymphatic obstruction

Diagnostic Evaluation

- History and physical exam: Assess for the presence of an underlying breast mass and involvement of axillary and supraclavicular nodes
    - A high index of suspicion for inflammatory cancer is necessary if a suspected breast infection does not rapidly improve with antibiotic administration
- Bilateral mammogram to detect underlying mass/calcifications and assess the contralateral breast
- Biopsy is indicated for any suspicious mammographic abnormalities or palpable masses
- All suspected cases of inflammatory breast cancer require a tissue diagnosis of the involved skin via a skin biopsy
- Metastatic workup is essential in all cases including a CBC, LFTs, bone scan, chest X-ray, and a CT scan of the chest, abdomen, and pelvis

Treatment/Management

- Once the diagnosis is confirmed, the patient is initially treated with systemic chemotherapy
- If clinical improvement occurs after 4–6 cycles of chemotherapy, surgery is undertaken (generally a modified radical mastectomy)
- Chemotherapy should again be given following surgery
    - Since this disease is so aggressive and traditional chemotherapies are only moderately effective, a taxane-based chemotherapy regimen is often added
- External beam radiation should be given after completion of chemotherapy to control local chest and chest wall disease

Prognosis/Complications

- 5-year survival is <5%
- Pre-operative chemotherapy followed by mastectomy and radiation has improved survival somewhat in recent years
- Local and/or chest wall recurrence occurs in 60% of cases

Skin Disease

JOHN J. RAVES, MD
BRIAN S. JU, MD

Section 7

58. Skin Anatomy, Facts, and Pearls

- The skin is the largest organ of the body
- The skin is approximately 1.2 mm thick, but varies from 0.5 to 6.0 mm
- The skin has three main levels:

Epidermis
- Includes the stratum corneum, supra basal layer, basal layer, Langerhan's cells, melanocytes, and basement membrane
- Outermost layer is the stratum corneum, consisting of non-viable, keratinized cells, which prevents loss of water, plasma, and electrolytes
- Innermost layer is the basal layer (stratum germinativum), which contains melanocytes and keratin-producing cells
- Epidermal appendages include the nails, hair, sebaceous glands, and sweat glands
- The epidermis replaces itself about every 4 weeks

Dermis
- Thin, superficial layer (papillary dermis)
- Thicker, deep layer (reticular dermis) that includes blood vessels, fibroblasts, and the termination of most of the epidermal appendages (e.g., sweat glands, hair follicles)

Subcutanteous Fat
- Blood vessels
- Adipose tissue

Functions of the Skin
- Thermal regulation, through eccrine sweat glands and vasodilation and vasoconstriction of vessels
- Secretion of sweat
- Sensory organs, including temperature, pain, and touch
- Protective barrier against environmental and bacterial invasion

Primary Lesions
- Macule: Flat, circumscribed lesion that differs in color or appearance from the surrounding skin
- Papule: Elevated lesion usually <0.5 cm in diameter
- Pustule: Raised lesion with purulent content
- Patch: Area of skin that differs from the surrounding skin; usually >1 cm in diameter
- Plaque: Broad, flat, elevated lesion usually >1 cm in diameter
- Nodule: Round or dome-shaped, solid lesion larger than 1 cm in diameter
- Tumor: Solid lesion similar to nodule, but larger than 2 cm in diameter
- Vesicle: Elevated lesion containing fluid, usually <1 cm in diameter; usually tense
- Bulla: Elevated lesion containing fluid, usually >1 cm in diameter; may be tense or flaccid
- Cyst: Spherical or oval nodule containing fluid or semi-solid material
- Rash: A very general term that indicates a change in the epidermis; may have many different appearances
- Wheal: Pale, pink or red, elevated plaque or papule that disappears within hours (characteristic of hives)
- Erosion: Depressed lesion resulting from loss of epidermis without involvement of dermis
- Ulcer: Depressed lesion resulting from loss of epidermis and a portion of dermis
- Scar: A hard, sclerotic area of skin due to damage to the dermis with subsequent healing
- Excoriation: Superficial excavations of skin due to scratching
- Fissure: Linear cracks in the skin; may be painful
- Telangiectasia: Dilated, small blood vessels (capillaries, venules, or arterioles)

Secondary Changes
- Erythema: Redness of skin, often accompanied by increased temperature, pain, and swelling
- Hyperpigmentation: Increase in skin pigment, resulting in darker area of skin
- Hypopigmentation: Decrease in skin pigment, resulting in lighter area of skin
- Hyperkeratosis: Thickening of stratum corneum
- Atrophy: Loss of dermis and/or subcutaneous fat
- Exudate: Skin fluid in areas of inflammation, lesions, or surgical sites; may be clear, cloudy, or purulent
- Crust: Accumulation of dried exudate
- Scale: Shedding of outer layer of epidermis (stratum corneum)
- Lichenfication: Thickened plaques from repeated rubbing or scratching of skin
- Purpura: Ecchymotic (dark purple), non-blanching skin lesions from vascular injury and hemorrhage

- Danger signs in moles include asymmetry, border irregularity, bleeding, color changes, increase in diameter, itching, or any other unusual changes

59. Hidradenitis Suppurativa

Etiology/Pathophysiology

- An infection of the apocrine glands, which may extend into adjacent tissues
- *Staphylococcus* and *Streptococcus* are common infectious agents
- Occurs in areas where apocrine glands are numerous: Axillae, groin, perineum, and perianal
- Etiology is unknown; associated with a blockage of the apocrine gland openings leading to chronic inflammation and infection
- More common in individuals with very curly hair, women (may be associated with menses), and patients with a family history
- Onset after puberty
- Excess perspiration is a risk factor (e.g., obese or athletic patient)
- May be associated with irritable bowel syndrome, Down's syndrome, Sjogren's syndrome, Herpes simplex, Graves' disease, arthritis

Differential Dx

- Cellulitis
- Infected sebaceous cyst
- Folliculitis
- Granuloma inguinale
- Lymphogranuloma venereum
- Pilonidal disease
- Tuberculosis

Presentation/Signs & Symptoms

- Tender, firm nodules and chronic infection in the axilla, inguinal area, or perineum is the most common complaint
- May see spontaneous purulent drainage
- Often recurrent
- Aggravated by heat, perspiration, poor hygiene, and obesity
- May progress to cellulitis
- May result in considerable scarring of the involved area(s)

Diagnostic Evaluation

- History and physical examination
- Culture of the drainage fluid
- If systemic symptoms are present, appropriate workup may include CBC and blood cultures

Treatment/Management

- Simple abscesses may respond to incision and drainage
- Antibiotics are indicated if cellulitis or fever is present
- Further surgical intervention may be required for refractory or complicated cases
    - Excision or curettage of the infected areas
    - Radical excision and skin graft in intractable disease
    - Laser and radiation treatments are being investigated
- Chronic antibiotic therapy (e.g., erythromycin, tetracyclines) may be indicated

Prognosis/Complications

- A chronic condition with frequent recurrences in other areas
- Healing of acute exacerbations usually occurs in 1–4 weeks
- Progression to scarring and tract formation may occur

60. Pilonidal Disease

Etiology/Pathophysiology

- A poorly understood condition associated with a hair-containing sinus in the buttock crease (midline sacrococcygeal region)
  - The exact etiology of this disease remains a puzzle
  - May be an acquired condition resulting from the ingrowth of a hair or hair follicle with subsequent cyst formation (also called a sinus) and inflammatory response
  - May become secondarily infected (*Staphylococcus aureus* and *Bacteroides* are the most common)
- Incidence of 25 cases per 100,000 people
- More common in males
- Usually occurs in the second to fourth decades of life
- Risk factors include male gender, obesity, family history, prolonged sitting, and trauma

Differential Dx

- Perianal abscess
- Carbuncle/furuncle
- Osteomyelitis
- Coccygeal sinus
- Sebaceous cyst
- Hidradenitis suppurativa
- Anal fistula
- Syphilis
- Tuberculosis

Presentation/Signs & Symptoms

- Midline gluteal (buttock) cleft tenderness
- May present as a subcutaneous fluctuant mass that represents abscess formation
  - Purulent drainage, swelling, induration, and erythema may be present
- A pore opening representing the sinus tract may be present on the midline gluteal skin
- In rare cases, systemic symptoms (e.g., fever) may be present
- Rectal exam is usually unremarkable

Diagnostic Evaluation

- A clinical diagnosis based on history and physical examination
  - Rectal exam is necessary to rule out perianal or perirectal disease
- Diagnostic tests are not indicated

Treatment/Management

- Asymptomatic patients may be observed
  - Ensure proper hygiene
  - Occasionally shaving the gluteal cleft area to remove hair may reduce recurrence
- Acute cases are treated with incision and drainage, wound packing, and strict hygiene
- Chronic or recurrent cases may require surgical excision
  - Elliptical excision with primary skin closure
  - Wide excision without primary skin closure (marsupialization)
  - Excision with local rotational skin flap

Prognosis/Complications

- 30–40% recur despite treatment
- Excision of midline pits after the initial drainage may reduce recurrence
- Other complications include further infection or abscess formation

61. Squamous Cell Carcinoma

Etiology/Pathophysiology

- A carcinoma of keratinocytes that occurs in skin and the mucosa of the mouth and anus
- The second most common type of skin cancer
- Associated with sun exposure, irritants, burns (Marjolin ulcer), scars, chronic ulcers, human papillomavirus infection, hydrocarbons, and radiation
- Appears on the ears, cheeks, lower lips, and back of hands
- Squamous cell carcinoma derived from sun-induced exposure rarely metastasizes; squamous cell carcinoma in immunocompromised patients has a more virulent course and may metastasize early

Differential Dx

- Other skin cancers (e.g., melanoma, basal cell carcinoma)
- Metastatic skin cancer
- Seborrheic keratosis
- Dermatofibroma
- Cherry hemangioma
- Benign nevi (e.g., blue nevus, halo nevus)

Presentation/Signs & Symptoms

- Often asymptomatic; however, bleeding, tenderness, or pain may be present
- Early lesions appear as firm, erythematous plaques or nodules with vague margins
- As lesions grow, they become raised and fixed and may ulcerate
- May be associated with aberrant keratinization and the production of cutaneous "horns"
- Leukoplakia may be present

Diagnostic Evaluation

- Biopsy is diagnostic
- Histology reveals malignant epithelial cells the extend into the dermis

Treatment/Management

- Treated by surgical excision
    - Primary closure for smaller defects
    - Skin grafting or flap reconstruction for larger lesions
- Given the poor prognosis of recurrent disease, every effort should be made to fully excise the tumor during the initial surgery
- Cryosurgery, curettage, and electrocautery can be used for small superficial lesions with low likelihood of nodal involvement
- Radiation is generally reserved for the elderly

Prognosis/Complications

- Most patients do well following surgical excision
- Overall cure rate is 90%
- Tumors in immunocompromised patients have a higher mortality rate secondary to the increased risk of metastasis
- Lip and ear tumors have much higher rate of recurrent and malignant disease

62. Basal Cell Carcinoma

Etiology/Pathophysiology

- Malignancy of the skin that probably arises from the pluripotent cells of the basal layer of the epidermis
- Characterized by slow, steady growth and rare metastasis, but local ulceration and tissue destruction may occur
- The most common type of skin cancer
- Associated with sun exposure, fair complexion, radiation exposure, arsenic, immunosupression, xeroderma pigmentosum, nevoid basal cell carcinoma syndrome, or prior history of non-melanoma skin cancer
- More common in men
- Often seen in the face and neck
- Usually found after age 40
- Subtypes include nodular ulcerative, superficial, and sclerosing

Differential Dx

- Benign nevi (e.g., blue nevus, halo nevus)
- Other skin cancers (e.g., melanoma, squamous cell carcinoma)
- Metastatic skin cancer
- Seborrheic keratosis
- Dermatofibroma
- Cherry hemangioma

Presentation/Signs & Symptoms

- Papular or nodular lesion with central erosion and waxy, pearly edges ("rodent ulcer")
- Telangiectasias are frequently visible within the lesion
- Bleeding or ulceration may occur (i.e., with minor trauma)
- 90% occur on the head and neck

Diagnostic Evaluation

- History and physical examination
- Biopsy is diagnostic

Treatment/Management

- Complete removal of the tumor via surgical excision with 1–2 mm margins is the gold standard
- Other treatment options include curettage, electrodessication, cryotherapy, and radiation
- Mohs' surgery (microscopic excision with tumor mapping) may be used in cosmetically sensitive areas

Prognosis/Complications

- Recurrent tumors are usually more aggressive than primary lesions
- Overall cure rates of low risk tumors are better than 90%, especially if Mohs' surgery is used

63. Malignant Melanoma

Etiology/Pathophysiology

- A malignancy of melanocytes
- The leading cause of skin cancer deaths
- Risk factors include sun exposure, multiple or dysplastic nevi, early life severe sunburn (especially in fair skinned individuals), age >60, large numbers of moles, family history, xeroderma pigmentosum, and familial atypical mole melanoma syndrome
- Most types of melanoma extend radially, except for the nodular sclerosing type, which penetrates vertically into the subcutaneous tissues
- Metastasizes to the liver, lung, brain, bone, adrenal, heart, and bowel
- Superficial spreading is the most common type and has the best prognosis
    - Commonly occurs on the back and legs
- Lentigo maligna type occurs in sun-exposed areas
    - Primarily in the elderly (average age of diagnosis 70)
    - Slow growth; excellent prognosis
- Acral lentiginous type occurs primarily on the palms, soles, and nail beds and is more common in blacks
    - Usually large at the time of diagnosis
    - Very aggressive
- Nodular sclerosing type has rapid growth and is often fatal

Differential Dx

- Benign nevi (e.g., blue nevus, halo nevus)
- Other skin cancers (e.g., basal cell carcinoma, squamous cell carcinoma)
- Metastatic skin cancer
- Seborrheic keratosis
- Dermatofibroma
- Cherry hemangioma

Presentation/Signs & Symptoms

- Solitary lesion, most frequently on back or other sun-exposed areas
- Flat or raised macule/nodule
- Satellite pigmentation (due to local metastases) and erythema
- Ulceration and bleeding may suggest malignancy
- May arise in the skin, mucus membranes, CNS, nail beds (subungual melanoma), or eyes
- Men tend to have disease on the trunk and upper arm; women have disease on the extremities
- Patients should be examined for lymphadenopathy

Diagnostic Evaluation

- History and physical examination
    - Asymmetry: Asymmetric shape suggests malignancy
    - Border: Irregular or "smudged" borders suggest malignancy
    - Color: Non-uniform color suggests malignancy
    - Diameter: Lesions >5 mm tend to suggest malignancy
    - Enlargement: Lesions that appear to be changing in size or shape tend to be malignant
- Excisional biopsy is diagnostic for melanoma (punch biopsy is contraindicated)
- Full-body CT scan and laboratory studies may be indicated

Treatment/Management

- Wide surgical excision
    - Necessary margins depend on the depth of tumor penetration
    - For small depth, early lesions, the excisional biopsy may be sufficient
    - If depth of invasion is 1–4 mm, 2 cm margins of excision are indicated
    - If >4 mm, 2–3 cm margins with possible fascial resection may be necessary
- Lymph node dissection for palpable lymph nodes
- For non-palpable lymph nodes, sentinel node biopsy is indicated to evaluate for micrometastases
    - If positive, lymph node dissection is indicated
- Chemotherapy, interferon-β, and interleukin-2 are commonly indicated for metastases

Prognosis/Complications

- Metastatic disease to skin and/or internal organs is the most feared complication of melanoma (survival of 6–9 months)
- Prognosis is inversely related to the depth of invasion at diagnosis (Breslow's classification)

<0.76 mm	99% 5-year survival
0.76-1.49	85% 5-year survival
1.5-2.49	84% 5-year survival
2.5-3.99	70% 5-year survival
>4	44% 5-year survival
Metastases	<10% 5-year survival

- History of melanoma dramatically increases the risk of a second primary lesion

64. Benign Skin Lesions

Etiology/Pathophysiology

- Seborrheic keratosis is the most common benign skin tumor; usually found in the elderly with long-term sun exposure; no malignant potential
- Verrucae (common warts) are caused by human papillomavirus
- Epidermal inclusion cysts (sebaceous cyst) are layers of epidermal cells filled with epithelial debris and sebum; may become infected
  - Often occurs in scalp, face, ears, neck, and back
- Dermoid cyst is deeper than sebaceous cysts; may extend to bone, meninges
- Hidradenomas are firm, discrete, mobile benign sweat gland tumors found in labial or perirectal regions
- Pigmented nevi (junctional, intradermal, compound, blue, spindle cell, and giant hairy nevi) are melanocyte-containing cells that produce melanin
  - Risk of malignancy is increased in junctional and giant nevi
- Keratoacanthoma is premalignant, locally destructive, and grows rapidly
  - Squamous cell carcinoma may be found in up to 25% of lesions
- Solar (actinic) keratosis is a premalignancy occurring in sun-exposed areas
  - Squamous cell carcinoma develops in 20% of cases
- Bowen's disease is a squamous cell carcinoma in situ
- Leukoplakia is a premalignant lesion that occurs on oral or rectal mucosa or the vulva

Differential Dx

- Differentiate from malignant tumors (malignant melanoma, basal cell carcinoma, squamous cell carcinoma)
- Psoriasis
- Eczema

Presentation/Signs & Symptoms

- Seborrheic keratosis: Waxy, dry, flat, brown pigmented lesions
- Epidermal inclusion cysts: Usually elevated and filled with a foul smelling caseous material; often occur in scalp, face, ears, neck, and back
- Keratoacanthomas may grow up to 4 cm in diameter with a horn-filled center
- Solar (actinic) keratosis is a rough, scaly epidermal lesion
- Bowen's disease presents as a well-defined reddened plaque with an adherent yellow crust
- Leukoplakia appears as a raised whitish lesion on oral or rectal mucosa or the vulva

Diagnostic Evaluation

- History and physical examination
- Biopsy is diagnostic and usually therapeutic

Treatment/Management

- Most lesions are left alone or treated by excision
- Seborrheic keratosis: Cryotherapy or shave excision
- Warts: Electrodessication or cryotherapy; avoid surgical excision as the virus may spread throughout the wound; may resolve spontaneously
- Nevi are usually observed; junctional and giant nevi are excised due to risk of melanoma
- Keratoacanthoma: May be observed for a short time in anticipation of spontaneous disappearance; persistent lesions should be excised due to risk of malignant transformation
- Actinic keratosis, Bowen's disease, and leukoplakia should all be excised to avoid malignancy

Prognosis/Complications

- Most lesions are benign and curable
- Premalignant lesions require excision to rule out malignancy

65. Burns

Etiology/Pathophysiology

- Thermal, electrical, or chemical injury resulting in damage to the skin barrier, inflammation and cellular damage/death, and systemic immunosuppresion
- Loss of skin integrity results in increased insensible fluid losses, impaired thermoregulation, and increased risk of infection
  - Fluid is rapidly lost due to disrupted skin and third-spacing into the interstitium of damaged tissues
  - Infection is often due to *Staphylococcus, Streptococcus*, and *Pseudomonas*
- Smoke inhalation injury is often associated with burns, resulting in acute lung injury with bronchospasm, airway and airspace edema, pneumonitis, and eventually ARDS
  - May also result in carbon monoxide or hydrogen cyanide poisoning
  - Facial burns, singed nose hair or eyebrows, voice changes, and carbonaceous sputum suggest upper airway injury
- Skin has two layers: Epidermis and dermis; the dermis contains nerves and blood supply; full thickness burns destroy nerves at this level

Differential Dx

- Thermal burns
- Chemical burns
  - Acid burns cause coagulation necrosis, which limits the depth of penetration
  - Alkali burns (e.g., lye, lime, cement) cause liquefaction necrosis, resulting in deep penetration with systemic effects
- Electrical burns (including lightning)
- Child abuse
- Scalded skin syndrome

Presentation/Signs & Symptoms

- First-degree (epidermis only)
  - Resembles sunburn
  - Erythema, pain, no blistering or scar
- Second-degree (partial thickness)
  - Dermis is involved
  - Pain, redness, and blistering
- Third-degree (full thickness)
  - Pain-free due to destruction of nerve endings
  - White pearly appearance due to absent blood flow
  - Visible thrombosed vessels are pathognomonic
- Fourth-degree: Burn of muscle or bone
- Monitor for circumferential burns of the extremities or chest

Diagnostic Evaluation

- Estimate burn size by "rule of 9s" to guide therapy and need for transfer to burn center
  - Each arm 9%   Anterior torso 18%   Head/neck 9%
  - Each leg 18%   Posterior torso 18%   Perineum 1%
- Minor burn: <15% of total body surface area (TBSA)
- Moderate burn: 15–25% of TBSA
- Major burn: >25% of TBSA; full-thickness burns covering >10% of TBSA; burns of the hand, face, or perineum; circumferential burns of the chest or extremities; inhalation injury; or deep electric burn
- Labs may include CBC, electrolytes, renal function, ABG, carboxyhemoglobin level, alcohol and toxicology screens
- Chest X-ray in cases of inhalation injury may show pulmonary edema or ARDS
- Burn wound infection is diagnosed by wound culture or biopsy that demonstrates >10^5 organisms

Treatment/Management

- Prompt attention to airway, breathing, and circulation
  - Airway edema may compromise breathing—early intubation if evidence of inhalation injury, significant facial or neck burns, or respiratory distress
- Aggressive fluid administration to replace insensible losses is the most important aspect of resuscitation
  - Many formulas (e.g., Parkland) are available to estimate fluid requirements; resuscitate as necessary to maintain adequate urine output (50 cc/hr)
- Pain control, IV antibiotics, and tetanus prophylaxis
- Transfer to a burn center is necessary for patients with smoke inhalation, electrical burns, >20% of body surface involved, or second-degree burns to hands, feet, face, or perineum
- Circumferential extremity burns may require escharotomy or fasciotomy for vascular compromise
- Circumferential burns to the neck or chest require escharotomy if respiratory compromise occurs

Prognosis/Complications

- First-degree burns heal within a week
- Superficial second-degree heal in 1–3 wks
- Deep second-degree and third-degree often require skin grafting to prevent scarring
- Complications include infection, inhalation injury, carbon monoxide or cyanide poisoning, hypothermia, and eschar formation
- 50% of deaths occur due to inhalation injury
- Topical antibiotics are usually applied, including bacitracin (partial thickness), silver sulfadiazine, mafenide acetate, and silver nitrate
  - Silver sulfadiazine may result in neutropenia
  - Mafenide may cause metabolic acidosis
  - Silver nitrate may cause hyponatremia

Hernias

Section 8

JOHN J. RAVES, MD
BRIAN S. JU, MD

66. Hernia Anatomy, Facts, and Pearls

- A hernia is a weakness or disruption in the fibromuscular tissue (fascia or muscle) of the abdominal wall, resulting in a protrusion of abdominal contents (peritoneum, fat, omentum, and/or abdominal viscera)
- In general, most hernias should be repaired to avoid complications (incarceration, strangulation, ischemia, perforation, bowel obstruction, pain)
- The size of the abdominal wall defects through which the hernia protrudes predicts the risk for strangulation: Smaller defects are *more* likely to result in strangulation than larger defects

Definitions of Terms

- Hernia sac: As the peritoneum protrudes through the abdominal wall defect, it is referred to as a hernia sac; it may contain only pre-peritoneal fat or abdominal contents
- Reducible: Hernia can be replaced (e.g., by manual reduction, by lying down) to its proper anatomic location
- Incarceration (or irreducible): The hernia sac and/or organs contained within the sac cannot be reduced back into the abdominal cavity; may or may not cause bowel obstruction or ischemia of the herniated abdominal contents
- Strangulation: Compromised blood flow to the contents of the hernia sac (viscera or omentum), resulting in ischemia, perforation, or gangrene; usually associated with an incarcerated hernia
- Ventral hernia: Any hernia involving the anterior abdominal wall; usually excludes inguinal hernias
- Indirect inguinal hernia: Herniation through the internal inguinal ring, lateral to Hasselbach's triangle and the inferior epigastric vessels
- Direct inguinal hernia: Herniation through or within Hasselbach's triangle, medial to the inferior epigastric vessels
- Hasselbach's triangle is bordered by the inferior epigastric vessels, the lateral border of the rectus sheath, and the inguinal ligament
- The inguinal ligament extends from the anterior superior iliac spine to the pubic tubercle and is derived from the external oblique muscle
- Femoral hernia: Herniation into the femoral canal, below the inguinal ligament
- Umbilical hernia: Herniation through midline fascia at the umbilicus
- Epigastric hernia: Herniation through midline fascia above the umbilicus
- Spigelian hernia: Herniation below the arcuate line, lateral to the rectus abdominis
- Incisional hernia: Herniation through a wound closure site
- Sliding hernia: The protruding hernia sac is partly formed by a retroperitoneal organ (e.g., bladder, sigmoid colon, cecum)
- Littre's hernia: Any hernia that contains a Meckel's diverticulum
- Richter's hernia: Incarceration of only one side of the bowel wall; this herniated portion of the bowel may strangulate and become necrotic without resulting in bowel obstruction
- Pantaloon hernia: A combined direct and indirect inguinal hernia that "straddles" the inferior epigastric vessels

67. Ventral Hernias

Etiology/Pathophysiology

- Ventral hernias occur through a defect in the anterior abdominal wall
- Incisional hernia: Weakness or defect in the abdominal wall that occurs at a site of prior surgical incision
  - Most common type of ventral hernia
  - Roughly 5% of abdominal surgical procedures result in incisional hernias
  - Risk factors include inadequate fascial closure, wound infection, midline incision, obesity, pregnancy, ascites, malnutrition, elderly, peritoneal dialysis, steroids, and chemotherapy
  - Parastomal hernias may occur at the site of an ileostomy or colostomy
- Epigastric hernia: Herniation through a defect in the linea alba above the umbilicus
  - More common in men
  - May be multiple
- Rectus diastasis: An acquired widening of the linea alba (the fusion of the aponeuroses of the rectus abdominis sheaths) resulting in bulging of the linea alba, mimicking an epigastric hernia
- Spigelian hernia: Occurs at the lateral edge of the rectus abdominis below the umbilicus at the semicircular line of Douglass
- Umbilical: A type of ventral hernia that occurs at the umbilicus (see associated "Umbilical Hernias" entry)

Differential Dx

- Rectus diastasis
- Soft tissue mass or tumor
- Fluid collection (e.g., hematoma) at prior operative site

Presentation/Signs & Symptoms

- Bulge in the abdominal wall
- The clinician may be able to feel the fascial edge of the defect upon palpation of the hernia
- May or may not be reducible
- May present with signs of obstruction and pain if bowel contents are incorporated into the hernia
- Incisional hernia: Mass or bulging at or near a surgical scar or a stoma site (ileostomy or colostomy)
- Epigastric: Midline mass or bulging between the xiphoid process and the umbilicus
- Spigelian hernia: Mass or bulging below the umbilicus at the lateral edge of the rectus muscle

Diagnostic Evaluation

- Physical exam with detection of an abdominal wall mass or bulge is usually diagnostic
- CT scan may be necessary, especially in obese individuals
- Abdominal X-ray may be ordered if suspect bowel obstruction
  - Obstruction presents with dilated loops of small bowel with air-fluid levels proximal to the obstruction and absence of gas distal

Treatment/Management

- All ventral hernias require surgical repair
  - Elective repair of unobstructed hernias
  - Elective repair may be delayed if necessary (e.g., weight loss in obese patients, cessation of tobacco use) to prevent complications
  - Repair of incisional hernias is delayed until patients have recovered from their initial surgery
  - Emergent repair may be necessary if signs of obstruction or peritonitis are present
- Simple suture repair may be adequate for small incisional hernias if the fascial edges can be brought together without significant tension
- Mesh insertion may be necessary to prevent recurrence of the hernia and/or to close a wide abdominal hernia defect
- Laparoscopic approaches may be used in select cases for lysis of adhesions, reduction of the hernia sac, and insertion of mesh

Prognosis/Complications

- The most frequent complication is recurrence of the hernia (even with optimal technique)
- Wound infection, adhesions, and chronic pain may also occur
- Wound infection may require removal of mesh, if present

68. Inguinal Floor Hernias

Etiology/Pathophysiology

- 75% of abdominal hernias are inguinal hernias
- Inguinal hernias include indirect inguinal (most common), direct inguinal, and femoral
  - All inguinal hernias are more common on the right side
  - Direct and indirect hernias are more common in males
  - Femoral hernias are more common in females and common in pregnancy
- Indirect inguinal hernia: The hernia sac penetrates "indirectly" through the internal ring of the inguinal canal with the spermatic cord, lateral to the epigastric vessels
  - May be congenital or acquired (occurs any time from infancy to old age)
  - Congenital cases are often due to incomplete obliteration of the processus vaginalis (more common in premature infants)
- Direct inguinal hernia: The hernia sac penetrates "directly" through the floor of the inguinal canal (Hasselbach's triangle), medial to the epigastric vessels
  - Due to an acquired abdominal wall weakness (e.g., elderly, activity)
  - Commonly associated with straining, heavy lifting, and coughing
- Femoral hernia: Occurs under the inguinal ligament medial to the femoral vessels and in the femoral triangle
  - Femoral hernias are the most prone to strangulation

Differential Dx

- Any condition that presents as an inguinal mass or groin pain must be considered in the differential
- Muscle strain
- Adenitis
- Epididymitis
- Testicular torsion
- Hidradenitis
- Lipoma
- Hematoma
- Varicocele
- Hydrocele
- Abscess
- Neoplasm
- Lymphoma
- Sebaceous cyst
- Ectopic testes

Presentation/Signs & Symptoms

- Mass or bulging in the inguinal region
  - May or may not be reducible
  - May or may not be tender to palpation
- Most inguinal hernias are without pain
- Symptomatic patients may have pain at rest and/or during strenuous activity
- Worsening pain or toxic symptoms must raise concern for a strangulated hernia

Diagnostic Evaluation

- Physical examination is often diagnostic
  - Patients should be examined when standing and lying
  - Valsalva maneuver (e.g., cough) may accentuate the protrusion of the hernia
  - If a bulge is felt below the inguinal canal, suspect a femoral hernia
- Ultrasound may be used to differentiate a hernia versus a solid groin mass
- CT scan may be necessary, especially in obese individuals

Treatment/Management

- In general, all inguinal hernias require surgical repair due to risk of enlargement, incarceration, and strangulation
  - The goal of repair is to reduce the hernia back into the abdominal cavity and repair the fascial defect
  - Open or laparoscopic procedures may be used
  - Repair options include suturing of the defect, placement of a mesh barrier to cover the defect, or placement of a mesh "plug" to fill the defect
- Gentle manual reduction of incarcerated hernias may be attempted with or without analgesia or sedation
- Emergent repair is necessary for strangulated hernias or incarcerated hernias that cannot be manually reduced
  - Direct visualization of the strangulated bowel during hernia repair is necessary to determine viability of the bowel

Prognosis/Complications

- Recurrence may be associated with repair under tension, a missed indirect hernia, or progressive fascial weakening
- Recurrent hernias are more prone to incarceration or strangulation
- Recurrence rates for inguinal hernias are 4–7%
  - Higher frequency of recurrence for direct hernias, given the poor inguinal floor tissue
  - Wound infection is a common cause of recurrent hernias

69. Umbilical Hernias

Etiology/Pathophysiology

- A midline fascial defect found at the umbilicus, allowing herniation of the peritoneum
- Often present in newborns
  - More common in black, female, and premature newborns
  - As the child grows, the umbilical ring usually closes by age 2
  - <5% of defects persist to adulthood
  - If the fascial defect is >1.5 cm, it rarely spontaneously closes
- In adults, umbilical hernias are thought to be acquired
  - Associated with ascites, pregnancy, and obesity
  - Umbilical hernias in adults have a high risk of incarceration with subsequent strangulation

Differential Dx

- Soft tissue mass or tumor
- Ventral hernia
- Incisional hernia

Presentation/Signs & Symptoms

- Umbilical or periumbilical mass
- Most cases are asymptomatic
  - The hernia sac (the "bulge") may be reducible or non-reducible
  - Some incarcerated (non-reducible) umbilical hernias may be asymptomatic
- Localized pain and tenderness over the hernia sac, without associated obstructive symptoms, suggests herniation of omentum (without bowel involvement) into the hernia sac
  - Severe pain without obstructive symptoms or generalized abdominal findings suggests infarcted omentum
- Signs of bowel obstruction or generalized abdominal pain may suggest that the small bowel is herniated

Diagnostic Evaluation

- Physical exam with detection of an umbilical mass or bulge is usually diagnostic
- CT scan may be necessary, especially in obese individuals
- Abdominal X-ray may be ordered if suspect bowel obstruction
  - Obstruction presents with dilated loops of small bowel with air-fluid levels proximal to the obstruction and absence of gas distal

Treatment/Management

- Pediatric umbilical hernias usually spontaneous close by age 2
  - Repair is usually delayed until age 4–5 to allow for potential spontaneous closure, unless significant symptoms are present
  - Larger defects (>1.5 cm) are less likely to close spontaneously, and operative repair is likely
- Nearly all umbilical hernias in adults should be repaired, even if asymptomatic and reducible
  - Patients with ascites (particularly cirrhotic patients with ascites) should not undergo umbilical hernia repair unless their ascites is well controlled or the overlying skin has become necrotic
- Simple, primary closure of the defect is usually sufficient

Prognosis/Complications

- Prognosis is excellent with very low rates of recurrence or postoperative complications
- Umbilical hernia repair should be avoided in cirrhotic patients with ascites due to an increased risk of recurrence and strong likelihood of infection of the ascitic fluid

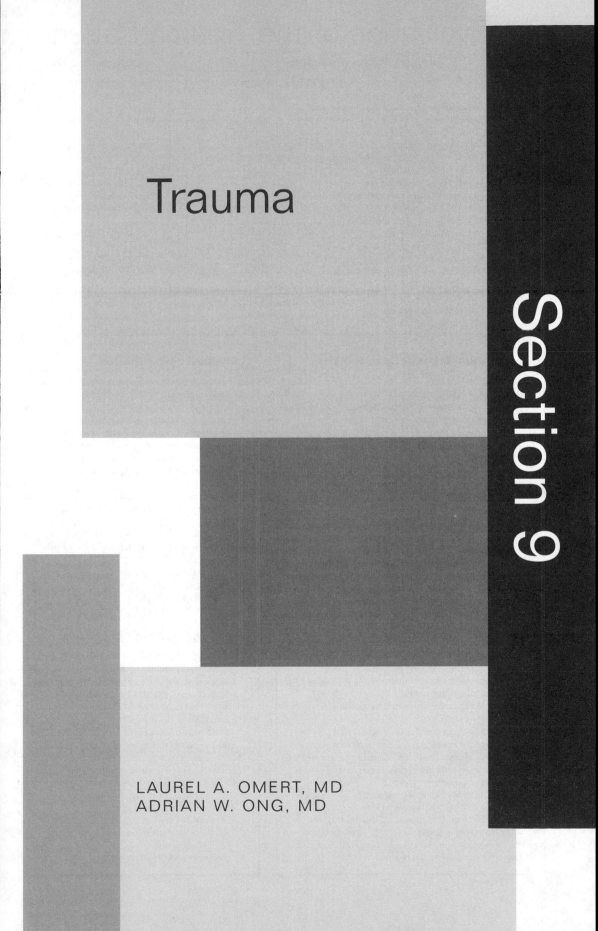

Trauma

Section 9

LAUREL A. OMERT, MD
ADRIAN W. ONG, MD

70. Evaluation of the Trauma Patient

Etiology/Pathophysiology

- Trauma often affects the young and can result in a lifetime of impairment
- Multi-step patient evaluation to rapidly identify life-threatening injuries
- Treatment begins in the field with pre-hospital care
- Life saving procedures (intubation, needle thoracostomy, spinal stabilization, fluid administration) should be performed prior to transport
- Primary survey: Airway, breathing, circulation, disability (neurologic status), and exposure/environment (completely disrobe patient and maintain body temperature with warm blankets)
- Secondary survey: Comprehensive head-to-toe physical exam
- Transfer to a designated trauma center may be necessary
- Unique challenges in trauma of children, elderly, and pregnant patients
- Pregnancy: Even minor trauma may cause placental abruption and fetal death; physiologic changes during pregnancy (e.g., 20% increase in pulse, 50% increase in blood volume) may mask early signs of shock; uterine blood flow is compromised before maternal hypotension occurs
- Elderly: May not tolerate even minor injuries due to poor reserve; may not be able to ↑ heart rate due to meds (e.g., β-blockers) or heart disease
- Pediatrics: Children have a large physiologic reserve; thus, they may appear stable but then rapidly decompensate
- See also "ATLS appendix"

Differential Dx

- Penetrating trauma: Gunshots, knives, impaled objects
- Blunt trauma (occurs due to organ compression, direct trauma, or deceleration injury): Motor vehicle or motorcycle crashes, falls, pedestrian accidents, assaults
- Trauma secondary to medical or environmental events
  - Seizure or MI that leads to a fall or a car accident
  - Burn patients may have blunt trauma from falling, jumping out of a window, or blast effect

Presentation/Signs & Symptoms

- Penetrating trauma
  - Gunshot wounds: Note type of weapon (e.g., shotgun versus handgun), velocity of weapon (high versus low), and distance from victim to weapon
  - Knife wounds: Examine for number and location of wounds, brisk bleeding, and evisceration
  - Impaled objects: Never remove in the field or emergency department
- Blunt trauma has a variable presentation
  - Note mechanism of injury (e.g., fall from significant height, sudden deceleration injury)
  - Always maintain a high index of suspicion for internal organ trauma

Diagnostic Evaluation

- In penetrating trauma, determine whether the knife or bullet entered a body cavity or remained in the subcutaneous tissue or fat
  - Examine clinically for entrance and exit wounds
  - Assess by radiographs for retained bullets or fragments
  - Impaled objects should only be removed in the operative room—never remove in the field or ED
- Blunt trauma is often subtle and thus requires a thorough physical exam and diagnostic studies
  - FAST ultrasound (Focused Abdominal Sonographic Test) should be performed in all patients with suspected abdominal trauma
  - Initial imaging includes chest, pelvic, cervical X-rays
  - CT imaging of head, neck, chest, abdomen, and/or pelvis may be indicated
  - Diagnostic peritoneal lavage (DPL) to evaluate for intra-abdominal bleeding or intestinal perforation

Treatment/Management

- Administer supplemental O_2 and cardiac monitoring
- Protect C-spine in all trauma patients
- Airway: Assess for need for intubation (e.g., airway obstruction, inadequate airway)
- Breathing: Intubate for inadequate ventilation or oxygenation
  - Chest decompression (needle or chest tube) is indicated for hemothorax or pneumothorax
- Circulation: Hypotension is considered to be due to blood loss and hypovolemia until proven otherwise
  - Establish two large bore IVs
  - Draw blood for type and cross match
  - Replace volume with warmed IV fluids
  - Infuse O^- blood if unresponsive to 2 liters of fluids
  - Control external hemorrhage with direct pressure
- Definitive repair of major chest and abdominal injuries often requires operative intervention

Prognosis/Complications

- Deaths occur in a trimodal distribution
  - Early deaths (within minutes) are usually due to brain, spinal cord, or large vessel injury
  - Second peak of deaths (a few hours post-injury) occurs due primarily due to hemorrhage
  - Third peak of deaths (days to weeks after injury) occurs due to infection and sepsis
- If patient presents in shock (systolic BP <90) and respiratory distress, mortality approaches 75%
- Prognosis of traumatic cardiac arrest is poor
  - 10% survival for penetrating trauma
  - 0% survival for blunt trauma
  - In general, emergency room thoracotomy should be attempted in cases of traumatic cardiac arrest due to penetrating truncal trauma but not for blunt trauma

71. Head Trauma

Etiology/Pathophysiology

- Brain injuries are a significant cause of morbidity and mortality in trauma patients
- Patients present along a spectrum from normal physical exam with minimal underlying cognitive dysfunction to a vegetative state
- Primary injury occurs at the time of trauma
- Secondary injury occurs after the initial insult due to hypoperfusion (i.e., hypotension, increased ICP), hypoxia, hyperglycemia, or anemia
- Intracranial hemorrhage can occur into the epidural space, subdural space (acute or chronic), subarachnoid space, or intraparenchymal tissue
- Head trauma from penetrating injury (usually gunshot wounds) occurs due to the physical path of the bullet plus associated concussive forces

Differential Dx

- Altered mental status
  - Drug/alcohol intoxication
  - Hypoglycemia
  - Seizure disorder
- Underlying neurologic condition
- Cervical spine or spinal cord injury

Presentation/Signs & Symptoms

- May present with headache, loss of consciousness, abnormal pupillary response, or other signs of intracranial hemorrhage
  - Unilateral pupil dilation suggests ipsilateral bleed with herniation
  - Bilateral pupil dilation suggests anoxic injury or bilateral herniation
- Battle's sign (mastoid ecchymosis), racoon eyes (orbital ecchymosis), and CSF rhinorrhea or otorrhea may signify a basilar skull fracture
- Signs of increased intracranial pressure include Cushing's reflex (hypertension, bradycardia, and hypopnea), decreasing level of consciousness, dilated pupils, and posturing (decorticate or decerebrate)

Diagnostic Evaluation

- Glasgow coma scale (eye opening, verbal response, motor response) is a simple and reproducible measure of mental status (scale ranges from 3–15)
  - Provides information on clinical course, prognosis, and treatment decisions (e.g., intubate if GCS <9)
  - GCS ≤8 indicates severe brain injury, 9–11 indicates moderate brain injury, and 12–15 indicates mild brain injury
- Head CT should be performed expeditiously in all patients with suspected closed head injury (indicated by loss of consciousness, seizure, vomiting, amnesia, focal neurologic findings, skull fracture), or penetrating head trauma
  - Cerebral contusion: Intraparenchymal hyperdensity
  - Epidural hematoma: Convex hyperdensity
  - Subdural hematoma (acute): Concave hyperdensity
  - Subdural hematoma (chronic): Concave hypodensity
  - Traumatic subarachnoid: Blood in subarachnoid space

Treatment/Management

- Rapid intervention with particular attention to ABCs (airway, breathing, circulation) is necessary to minimize secondary brain injury
- Treat elevated ICP only if symptomatic
  - Sedate patient and elevate head of bed 30°
  - Brief hyperventilation may be performed acutely to cause cerebral vasoconstriction
  - Mannitol for osmotic diuresis and free radical scavenging
  - Surgical decompression of deteriorating patients via trephination (burr hole) or ventriculostomy
- Intracranial bleeds require seizure prophylaxis (e.g., phenytoin) and may require surgical drainage
- Check coagulation studies (PT/PTT/INR) immediately and correct any coagulopathy to minimize intracranial bleeding
- Depressed skull fractures and penetrating trauma may require surgical repair

Prognosis/Complications

- Neurosurgical evaluation is required for any intracranial lesion
- Mortality increases with secondary brain injury
- One episode of SBP <90 doubles mortality
- 40% mortality if initial GCS <9
- Concussions may result in a post-concussive syndrome (vague, persistent symptoms such as headache, dizziness, and poor concentration) for weeks to months
- Patients with apparently normal presentation may have underlying cognitive deficits; neuropsychiatric testing is usually recommended

72. Neck Trauma

Etiology/Pathophysiology

- Neck structures susceptible to trauma include carotid/jugular/vertebral vessels, esophagus, pharynx, trachea, larynx, vertebrae, spine, spinal cord
- Penetrating neck trauma is generally due to stab or gunshot wounds
  - Management decisions are based on the involved neck zone
  - Zone I: Clavicles to cricoid cartilage
  - Zone II: Cricoid cartilage to angle of the mandible
  - Zone III: From angle of the mandible to base of the skull
- Blunt trauma may be due to motor vehicle accident (MVA), "clothesline" injury (e.g., on motorcycle or snowmobile), direct blow, strangulation, or hanging
- Associated with vascular, esophageal, and laryngotracheal injury
- Blunt vascular injury may cause carotid dissection or pseudoaneurysm formation with vessel thrombosis or occlusion
- Strangulation may result in vertebral and spinal cord injury, soft tissue trauma, vascular injury, or airway occlusion

Differential Dx

- Vascular injury to the carotid or vertebral arteries or jugular vein
- Nervous system injury (cranial nerves, spinal cord, autonomic nerves)
- Esophageal injury
- Laryngotracheal injury (vocal cord damage, cartilage fracture, recurrent laryngeal nerve)
- C-spine injury
- Intrathoracic injury

Presentation/Signs & Symptoms

- Airway injury: Dyspnea, stridor, hoarseness, hemoptysis, air bubbles from the wound, subcutaneous air, tracheal deviation
- Vascular injury: Active bleeding, bruit, hematoma (may compromise airway)
- Neurologic symptoms of carotid injury: Horner's syndrome, CVA/TIA with motor or sensory deficits
- Arterial or esophageal injuries may be asymptomatic
- Intrathoracic structures may be involved in lower neck trauma (e.g., subclavian vessels, lung)

Diagnostic Evaluation

- CT scan or plain films are used to evaluate blunt neck trauma
  - Lateral neck X-ray may reveal foreign body or airway impingement
  - C-spine X-rays are indicated to clear the C-spine
  - Chest X-ray may reveal thoracic involvement (e.g., pneumo/hemothorax, pneumomediastinum)
- Angiography is used to evaluate for vascular injury
  - Penetrating injury to Zones I or III require angiographic examination prior to operative exploration (due to the complex vascular anatomy of these zones)
  - Penetrating injuries to Zone II may be operatively explored or selectively managed with angiography, laryngo-tracheobronchoscopy, and esophagram/esophagoscopy
- Upper GI endoscopy or contrast study may be indicated to evaluate for upper esophageal injury

Treatment/Management

- Control of airway may be extremely difficult due to distorted anatomy and ongoing bleeding—intubation is indicated for any evidence of respiratory distress, large subcutaneous air, blood in the airway, or tracheal shift
- Control bleeding with direct pressure
- Immediate surgery is indicated if the patient is unstable or if there is obvious airway, esophageal, or vascular injury
- Penetrating neck trauma: Local wound closure if platysma has not been penetrated; imaging should be done before surgical exploration for Zones I and III injuries; Zone II injuries may undergo immediate surgical management
- Blunt neck trauma: May require surgery for laryngeal or esophageal injury; systemic anticoagulation is often indicated for vascular injuries to prevent clot formation and embolization

Prognosis/Complications

- Blunt trauma may be asymptomatic despite significant pathology—consider observation in blunt injuries with significant mechanisms even in the presence of negative imaging
- Esophageal and arterial injuries may also initially be asymptomatic
- Missed esophageal injury may result in life-threatening infection of neck or mediastinum

73. Blunt Chest Trauma

Etiology/Pathophysiology

- Most multiple trauma patients will have some element of chest trauma
- Pulmonary contusion: Direct lung damage with alveolar hemorrhage
- Pneumothorax (PTX): Air in the pleural space causing lung collapse
- Tension pneumothorax: PTX with continued air leak into the pleural space, resulting in hemodynamic instability due to increasing intrapleural pressure, mediastinal shift, and decreased venous return
- Hemothorax: Blood in pleural space, often secondary to lung laceration
- Tracheobronchial injury: Laceration of the airway
- Diaphragmatic injury: A sudden increase in intra-abdominal pressure (e.g., steering wheel to abdomen), results in abdominal herniation into thorax
- Esophageal injury: May be iatrogenic or due to trauma
- Rib fractures are common (10–25% of trauma patients); may indicate associated underlying lung injury (e.g., pulmonary contusion, hemothorax)
- Flail chest: Multiple contiguous rib fractures resulting in free-floating ribs with paradoxical motion on respiration
- Aortic rupture usually occurs distal to origin of the left subclavian artery
- Cardiac contusion/rupture
- Pericardial tamponade

Differential Dx

- The mechanisms of injury that cause chest trauma may also result in significant head, spine, abdominal, and/or pelvic injury

Presentation/Signs & Symptoms

- Tenderness, abrasions, and/or bruising may suggest significant chest wall injury
- Crepitus of the chest wall
- Dyspnea suggests diaphragm rupture, lung contusion, or tracheobronchial injury
- Shock commonly occurs with tension pneumothorax and massive hemothorax; less common with pericardial tamponade
- Respiratory distress with unequal breath sounds associated with hypotension, distended neck veins, and/or tracheal deviation suggests a tension pneumothorax
- Lack of breath sounds with dullness to percussion suggests a significant hemothorax

Diagnostic Evaluation

- Chest X-ray, ECG, and continuous cardiac monitoring
  - A widened mediastinum on chest X-ray may indicate traumatic aortic rupture
  - Infiltrates on chest X-ray suggests pulmonary contusion
- Suspected aortic rupture requires further evaluation with angiography (gold standard), chest CT, or transesophageal echocardiography (TEE)
- Bronchoscopy may be indicated to evaluate injuries to the major bronchi if persistent pneumothorax (despite tube thoracostomy), large air leak (from chest tube), or pneumomediastinum are present
- Esophagoscopy and/or contrast swallow are usually required to evaluate for esophageal injury if pneumomediastinum is present
- Ultrasound may be used to assess for hemopericardium

Treatment/Management

- Suspected tension pneumothorax requires immediate decompression, without delay for chest X-ray
  - Needle catheter decompression should be done at the second intercostal space at the mid-clavicular line
  - Chest tube should then be inserted into the fourth–fifth intercostal space at the midaxillary line
- Hemo- or pneumothorax require chest tube insertion
- Pulmonary contusion is usually treated by supportive care only; mechanical ventilation may be required for significant hypoxia and respiratory distress
- Rib fractures are treated conservatively
  - Pain relief is necessary to minimize atelectasis and respiratory insufficiency
  - Thoracic epidural analgesia may be required if intravenous opiates/NSAIDs are inadequate
- Surgical intervention is required for injury to the aorta, bronchi, or esophagus and massive hemothorax, hemopericardium, or cardiac rupture

Prognosis/Complications

- The number of rib fractures may be an indicator of significant complications (e.g., pneumonia, acute respiratory distress syndrome) and increases in mortality
- Inadequately drained hemothorax may become infected (empyema), requiring surgical intervention
- Delayed diagnosis of aortic or esophageal injury significantly increases mortality
- In general, emergency room thoracotomy for blunt trauma (thorax or abdomen) with cardiac arrest should not be done as mortality is 100%

74. Blunt Abdominal Trauma

Etiology/Pathophysiology

- Blunt abdominal trauma most commonly occurs due to motor vehicle crashes, struck pedestrians, falls, or assaults
- Mechanisms of blunt injury include deceleration and crush injury to solid organs and intestine
  - Injury to solid organs (e.g., liver, spleen, kidney) results in hemorrhage
  - Injury to intestine, resulting in perforation and peritonitis, occurs less commonly in blunt trauma
- Most commonly injured organs in blunt trauma are the liver and spleen

Differential Dx

- Associated injuries
  - Thoracic injury (lung, heart, or esophagus)
  - Diaphragmatic injury
  - Genitourinary injury
  - Pelvic fracture
  - Rib fracture

Presentation/Signs & Symptoms

- Pain is a good indicator of injury; however, lack of pain on abdominal exam does not reliably rule out intra-abdominal injury
- Hemodynamic instability or shock may be the only sign of abdominal trauma
- Peritonitis indicates an acute abdominal process that requires surgical intervention
- "Seatbelt sign": A red mark across the abdomen is a warning sign for possible intestinal injury
- Shoulder pain without obvious joint injury may indicate blood under the diaphragm

Diagnostic Evaluation

- Focused assessment with sonography for trauma (FAST exam) should be performed in all patients with suspected abdominal trauma to identify blood in the hepatorenal and splenorenal spaces, pelvis, and pericardium; however, will not identify the specific cause of bleeding
- Diagnostic peritoneal lavage (DPL) assesses for blood in the peritoneal cavity, but does not identify involved organ or evaluate retroperitoneum
  - Positive if gross blood or fluid lavage with >100,000 RBCs, >500 WBCs, fecal matter, or increased amylase
- Abdominal CT is indicated in stable patients to identify specific organ injuries and evaluate the retroperitoneum (for retroperitoneal bleeding and kidney or pancreas injury)
- MRI is the test-of-choice for diaphragm injuries
- Chest X-ray may reveal free abdominal air or ruptured diaphragm

Treatment/Management

- Unstable patients or those with clear signs of intra-abdominal injury (e.g., peritoneal signs on exam, diaphragmatic injury, abdominal free-air, evisceration) should immediately proceed to the operating room
- Most spleen and liver injuries can be managed conservatively; however, patients should be admitted to ICU for close monitoring and serial Hb levels
  - Surgical intervention or angiographic embolization is indicated for severe injury or persistent bleeding
- Pancreatic injury is generally treated conservatively
  - If a transection of the pancreas is suspected, ERCP may delineate whether major ductal disruption has occurred, requiring surgical resection
- Diaphragm injuries require surgical repair
  - If diagnosed shortly after the traumatic event, abdominal approach should be used
  - Subtle injuries identified weeks or months later are better approached through the chest

Prognosis/Complications

- Liver: Complications include delayed hemorrhage into the peritoneum or biliary tree (hemobilia), abscess, or biloma
- Spleen: Complications include delayed rupture and pseudocyst or abscess formation
  - Patients who undergo splenectomy are at risk for overwhelming post-splenectomy infection (OPSI) by encapsulated organisms
  - Administer vaccines against *S. pneumonia, N. meningitides,* and *H. influenzae*
- Pancreas: Complications include abscess, pseudocyst formation, and fistulae

75. Penetrating Abdominal Trauma

Etiology/Pathophysiology

- Most commonly due to stab or gunshot wounds
- Liver and small bowel are the most commonly damaged organs as they are the largest space-occupying organs in the abdominal cavity
- Any gunshot wound to the torso or any penetrating wound from the nipple line to the gluteal crease has the potential for intra-abdominal injury
- May have associated chest, diaphragmatic, or retroperitoneal injury
- The likelihood for severe intra-abdominal injury requiring surgical intervention depends on the wounding agent and the hemodynamic status of the patient
    - Gunshot wounds nearly always require exploratory surgery to manage intraperitoneal injuries
    - Stab wounds may not penetrate the peritoneum and are often managed conservatively

Differential Dx

- Thoracic injury (lung, heart, or esophagus)
- Diaphragmatic perforation
- Genitourinary injury

Presentation/Signs & Symptoms

- Hemorrhage resulting in shock will present with hypotension, tachycardia, altered mental status, and cold, clammy skin
- Local tenderness at the wound site or diffuse tenderness and guarding with rebound suggest peritonitis
- Wound may show signs of bleeding, evisceration of an organ (e.g., intestines, omentum), or drainage of fecal or small bowel contents

Diagnostic Evaluation

- Most patients with gunshot wounds should proceed directly to surgery; if only an entrance wound is present, an A/P and lateral abdominal X-ray may be done to document the location of the bullet before proceeding to the operating room
- Patients with stab wounds who present with shock, peritonitis, evisceration, or drainage of fecal or intestinal contents should proceed directly to surgery
- Stable patients without the above presentations may undergo local wound exploration (LWE) to determine whether the stab wound has violated the peritoneum
- Ultrasound of the heart and chest X-ray should be done where possible

Treatment/Management

- Proceed to surgery under the indications discussed in the above "Diagnostic Evaluation" box
- In rare cases where there is low suspicion of intra-abdominal penetration (e.g., tangential trajectory of bullet), a diagnostic peritoneal lavage (DPL), laparoscopy, or triple-contrast CT scan may be utilized to further assess for peritoneal violation
- If local wound exploration (LWE) of stab wounds does not show penetration of the anterior fascia, the patient may be discharged
- If the fascia is penetrated on LWE, several options are available, including observation alone, DPL, diagnostic laparoscopy, or laparotomy

Prognosis/Complications

- Prognosis depends on the physiologic state of the patient on admission to the emergency room and the severity of injuries
- Mortality of abdominal gunshot wounds is 20–30%
- Mortality of abdominal stab wounds is very low

76. Genitourinary Trauma

Etiology/Pathophysiology

- Genitourinary (GU) injuries occur in up to 5% of trauma patients, with an increased incidence in children
  - Kidney injuries account for 80% of GU trauma
  - Other injuries to bladder, urethra, ureter, penis, testicles, prostate
  - Often associated with lumbar, sacral, and pelvic fractures
- GU trauma may occur due to blunt or penetrating trauma
  - In blunt trauma, GU injuries can be difficult to diagnose and require a high index of suspicion
- Any mechanism wherein the patient ends up in a "straddle position" should raise suspicion for GU involvement (e.g., bicycle crash, falling onto a beam)
- Grading of renal injuries (via imaging or surgical exploration) is necessary for clinical management
  - Grade I: Contusion or subcapsular hematoma without laceration
  - Grade II: Laceration <1 cm or nonexpanding retroperitoneal hematoma
  - Grade III: Laceration >1cm or collecting system rupture
  - Grade IV: Laceration extending to collecting system or a renal vascular injury (e.g., thrombosis, laceration)
  - Grade V: Shattered kidney or avulsed hilum

Differential Dx

- Flank pain secondary to blunt torso trauma must be differentiated from renal injury
- Free fluid without solid organ injury may indicate bladder rupture
- Non-visualization of a kidney on ultrasound or CT should never be assumed to be congenital absence, but rather a renal artery injury until proven otherwise
- Peri-renal fluid on the right side may be secondary to a duodenal injury

Presentation/Signs & Symptoms

- Clues to GU injury may include blood on undergarments, inability to void, poor rectal tone, abnormal prostate exam, rectal lacerations, blood at the penile meatus, perineal hematoma or ecchymosis, or buttock injury
- Hematuria is a non-specific indicator of GU injury
- Flank pain or ecchymosis suggests renal injury
- Blood at the urethral meatus, scrotal hematoma, and high riding prostate on rectal exam are pathognomonic for urethral injury
- Resistance to passage of a urinary catheter

Diagnostic Evaluation

- Urinalysis determines the need for further workup
  - Gross hematuria requires imaging and further workup
  - Microscopic hematuria (>5 RBC/hpf) requires further workup only if mechanism of trauma is significant (e.g., rapid deceleration injury, penetrating injury)
- CT scan with contrast will identify and grade renal injuries and also evaluate associated injuries
- Angiography is indicated to assess the renal vasculature if there is non-visualization of the kidney on CT
- If urethral injury is suspected, a retrograde urethrogram must be performed before inserting a Foley catheter
  - Small urinary catheter is placed into distal urethra and contrast is injected
  - Extravasation of contrast indicates urethral injury
- Cystogram is indicated if bladder rupture is suspected
- Inject 250 mL of contrast into bladder via Foley catheter
- Extravasation of contrast indicates bladder injury

Treatment/Management

- Penetrating GU trauma should undergo laparotomy
  - Further surgical exploration of the kidney is necessary if a peri-nephric hematoma is found
  - Ureteral lacerations require surgical repair
- Blunt GU trauma with extravasation of contrast outside Gerota's fascia should undergo laparotomy
- Patients with angiography showing vascular injury should undergo laparotomy
- Nephrectomy may be necessary for uncontrolled hemorrhage, vascular injury, grade V renal injury, or large urinary extravasation
- Intraperitoneal bladder rupture requires surgical repair; extraperitoneal tears can be managed with Foley catheter drainage and repeat cystograms
- Urethral injuries may be treated by placement of a suprapubic cystostomy tube, cystoscopic catheter placement, or direct surgical repair

Prognosis/Complications

- In general, GU injuries are not immediately life-threatening
- Upper urinary tract injuries may result in bleeding, delayed ureteral leakage with infection, urinoma, incontinence, fistula, or infected hematoma
- Increase in BUN/creatinine following trauma may indicate a missed renal injury
- Urethral injury may result in stricture or fistula formation
- Hypertension and kidney stones may occur later in life in <5% of patients with renal injury
- Urethral injuries may cause voiding difficulties, strictures, and erectile dysfunction

77. Pelvic Fractures

Etiology/Pathophysiology

- Pelvic fractures occur in 10% of blunt trauma patients
- 1–5% of patients with pelvic fractures will have significant resultant hemorrhage
    - Internal bleeding into the pelvis or retroperitoneum may occur without external signs
- Pelvic fractures should be suspected following high energy blunt trauma (e.g., ejection from vehicle, motorcycle crash, fall from significant height, industrial crush injury)
- Due to a rich vascular supply of venous plexuses and arterial vessels, hemorrhage is the primary cause of death in pelvic fractures (up to 6 liters of blood may be lost into the retroperitoneal and pelvic spaces)
- Pelvic fractures may result in significant genitourinary (GU) injury (e.g., bladder rupture, urethral injury)

Differential Dx

- Blunt abdominal trauma
- Hip or upper femur trauma
- Flank or lumbar trauma

Presentation/Signs & Symptoms

- Pain and instability with pressure on the pelvis, lower abdominal or pelvic tenderness, ecchymosis, and restricted hip joint movement may be present; however, there may be no external signs or symptoms of trauma
- The presence of blood on rectal exam, gross hematuria, or urethral meatal blood or scrotal hematoma may indicate associated pelvic fracture
- Open wound or laceration in the perineal area may indicate an open pelvic fracture
- 20–30% of patients with pelvic fractures will have associated intra-abdominal injuries
- Shock may occur from major hemorrhage

Diagnostic Evaluation

- Pelvis X-ray is mandatory in all multiple trauma patients to identify occult pelvic fractures
    - The fracture pattern seen on X-ray may be broadly classified into three groups, depending on the force vectors producing the injury: Antero-posterior compression, lateral compression, and vertical shear
    - In general, A/P compression and vertical shear fractures are associated with greater pelvic hemorrhage
- CT scan is indicated if plain films are unclear and/or to identify the extent of fractures; may also show retroperitoneal hemorrhage
- Objective evaluation to rule out intra-abdominal injury is essential (CT scan, DPL)
- If urinary tract injury is suspected, a retrograde urethrogram and/or retrograde cystogram should be done
- Patients with a physical exam suggesting rectal injury should undergo proctosigmoidoscopy

Treatment/Management

- Emergent management of significant intra-abdominal or intra-thoracic bleeding should take priority over pelvic hemorrhage
- Significant bleeding from a pelvic fracture must be treated aggressively by resuscitation including blood replacement, followed by pelvic angiography with embolization and/or external fixation
    - >90% success rate with angiographic embolization
- All pelvic fractures require orthopedic consultation
- Stable fractures can usually be treated conservatively; unstable fractures generally require operative repair

Prognosis/Complications

- Overall mortality may be as high as 25% due to associated injuries and hemorrhage (more common in unstable fractures)
- With improved multidisciplinary management protocols, the death rate from exsanguination has decreased substantially
- Complications may include hemorrhage, GU injury, acetabular/hip joint injury, fat embolism, ARDS, wound infection/sepsis, and pulmonary embolus

78. Overview of Shock

Etiology/Pathophysiology

- A physiologic state of inadequate circulation, resulting in insufficient tissue perfusion and oxygenation
- Organ dysfunction and damage (may be reversible or irreversible) occurs with prolonged lack of perfusion
- Hypovolemic shock: Decreased intravascular volume
- Cardiogenic shock: Decreased cardiac output
- Distributive shock: Loss of vasomotor tone results in inappropriate vasodilatation despite hypotension
- Septic (infectious) shock: Bacterial toxins cause decreased vascular tone
- Neurogenic shock: Head or spinal cord injury causes decreased vascular tone

Differential Dx

- Hypovolemic shock
  - Hemorrhage
  - Dehydration (e.g., diarrhea)
  - Extravascular fluid sequestration (third-spacing)
- Cardiogenic shock
  - Intrinsic (e.g., ischemia, LV dysfunction, valve disease)
  - Extrinsic (e.g., tamponade, PE, pneumothorax)
- Distributive shock
  - Septic shock
  - Neurogenic shock
- Hypoadrenal shock
- Anaphylaxis

Presentation/Signs & Symptoms

- Early signs include orthostatic hypotension, mild tachycardia, diaphoresis
- Late signs include hypotension, significant tachycardia and tachypnea, altered mental status
- Vasoconstriction (resulting in narrow pulse pressure and cool extremities) in hypovolemic and cardiogenic shock
- Vasodilatation (wide pulse pressure and warm extremities) in distributive shock
- Signs and symptoms of underlying disease may be apparent (e.g., fever due to infection, chest pain due to MI, pallor due to blood loss)

Diagnostic Evaluation

- Emergent diagnosis, supportive care, and treatment are essential
- Clinical recognition of inadequate organ perfusion (e.g., hypotension, tachycardia, decreased urine output, altered mental status)
- Initial studies include CBC, electrolytes, renal function, lactate level (elevated in tissue hypoperfusion), PT/PTT, ABG (measures degree of acidosis), and ECG
- Further workup as necessary depending on the type of shock (see individual shock pages)
- Swan-Ganz (pulmonary artery) catheter placement may help identify the type of shock and guide management

	Cardiac Output	CVP/wedge pressure	SVR
Hypovolemic	↓	↓	↑
Cardiogenic	↓	↑	↑
Neurogenic	↓	↓	↓
Septic	↑	↓	↓

Treatment/Management

- Airway, Breathing, and Circulation—secure the airway, administer supplemental O_2, establish two large-bore IVs, and type/cross match
- Re-establish adequate tissue perfusion
  - IV fluid administration is the initial treatment for all forms of shock (be careful in cases of cardiogenic shock as pulmonary edema can rapidly occur from fluid overload)
  - Choice of vasoactive agents depends on the type of shock (see individual shock pages)
- Determine the specific type of shock and treat underlying causes appropriately
  - Blood transfusion and surgery to control bleeding for hemorrhagic shock
  - Antibiotics and vasopressors for septic shock
  - IV fluids and vasopressors for neurogenic shock
  - Inotropes and treatment of underlying cause for cardiogenic shock

Prognosis/Complications

- Outcome depends on etiology and rapid restoration of adequate perfusion
- Continuously monitor for adequacy of resuscitation (e.g., stabilization of blood pressure, improvement of tachycardia, good perfusion on exam, resolution of acidosis, adequate urine output)
- Admit all patients to an intensive care unit
- Persistent oxygen deprivation quickly causes irreversible cellular injury
- Sequelae include ARDS, cardiac ischemia, shock liver, DIC, neurologic damage, and acute renal failure due to ATN

79. Hypovolemic (Hemorrhagic) Shock

Etiology/Pathophysiology

- Blood or fluid loss that overwhelms the body's compensatory mechanisms to maintain perfusion and oxygenation
- Hypovolemic shock includes hemorrhage and volume loss from vomiting, diarrhea, third-spacing of intravascular fluid, or burns
- Hemorrhage
  - Trauma: Pelvic fracture, long bone injury (especially femur), vascular injury, retroperitoneal hemorrhage, solid organ injury
  - GI bleeds: Upper and lower GI tract bleeding
  - Vascular: Ruptured aneurysm, arteriovenous malformation (AVM)
  - Reproductive tract losses: Miscarriage, ectopic pregnancy, placenta praevia, malignancy
- Dehydration/fluid loss (e.g., vomiting, diarrhea, inadequate intake)
- Third-space fluid losses (e.g., pancreatitis, burns, nephrotic syndrome, liver failure, bowel infarction)

Differential Dx

- Cardiogenic shock
  - Intrinsic (e.g., ischemia, valvular disease, LV dysfunction)
  - Extrinsic (e.g., tamponade, PE, pneumothorax)
- Distributive shock
  - Septic shock
  - Neurogenic shock
- Anaphylaxis
- Hypoadrenal shock

Presentation/Signs & Symptoms

- Based on degree of blood loss (decompensation occurs after 40% of blood volume is lost)
- Mild (<20% of blood volume lost): Cool extremities, poor capillary refill, and diaphoresis
  - Blood pressure and urine output are normal in mild blood loss
- Moderate (20–40%): Tachycardia, tachypnea, orthostasis, oliguria, and anxiety
- Severe (>40%): Hypotension, narrow pulse pressure, weak distal pulses, severe tachycardia, tachypnea, absent bowel sounds, and altered mental status (ranging from confusion to lethargy)

Diagnostic Evaluation

- Initial studies include CBC, electrolytes, renal function, lactate level (elevated in tissue hypoperfusion), PT/PTT, ABG (measures degree of acidosis), and ECG
- Increased BUN/creatinine ratio and hypernatremia
- Identify sources of bleeding via ultrasound, CT scan, diagnostic peritoneal lavage, and/or endoscopy
- Swan-Ganz catheter placement may help distinguish from other types of shock and guide management

	Cardiac Output	CVP/wedge pressure	SVR
Hypovolemic	↓	↓	↑
Cardiogenic	↓	↑	↑
Neurogenic	↓	↓	↓
Septic	↑	↓	↓

Treatment/Management

- Secure airway, establish two large-bore IVs, administer supplemental O_2 and type/cross match
- Volume resuscitation
  - Rapid infusion of IV fluids with normal saline or lactated Ringer's solution (no evidence has proven albumin solutions to be beneficial)
  - Emergent blood transfusion for hemorrhage (O⁻ blood)
- Replace electrolytes as necessary
- Clotting factors: Give fresh frozen plasma, platelets, or cryoprecipitate to correct coagulation abnormalities
- Definitive control of bleeding may be indicated via angiographic embolization, endoscopic repair, and/or surgical intervention

Prognosis/Complications

- Outcome depends on etiology and rapid restoration of adequate perfusion
- Continuously monitor for adequacy of resuscitation (e.g., stable blood pressure, improvement of tachycardia, adequate perfusion on exam, resolution of acidosis, and adequate urine output)
- Admit all patients with shock to an ICU
- Persistent oxygen deprivation quickly causes irreversible cellular injury
- Sequelae include ARDS, cardiac ischemia, shock liver, DIC, neurologic damage, and acute renal failure due to ATN

80. Distributive Shock

Etiology/Pathophysiology

- Hypoperfusion due to a loss of vasomotor tone, resulting in inappropriate vasodilatation despite hypotension
- Vasodilatation increases the intravascular space; thus, the normally adequate intravascular volume is distributed throughout a much greater space, resulting in inadequate effective circulating volume
- Neurogenic shock is caused by blunt or penetrating trauma to the brain and/or spinal cord—CNS injury impairs sympathetic output, resulting in bradycardia, arterial and venous dilatation, and hypotension
- Septic shock is caused by overwhelming microbial infection that results in hypotension and hypoperfusion despite adequate fluid resuscitation

Differential Dx

- Cardiogenic shock
  - Intrinsic (e.g., ischemia, LV dysfunction, valve disease)
  - Extrinsic (e.g., tamponade, PE, pneumothorax)
- Hypovolemic shock
  - Hemorrhage
  - Dehydration
  - Third-spacing
- Anaphylaxis
- Hypoadrenal shock

Presentation/Signs & Symptoms

- Hypotension
- Wide pulse pressure
- Warm extremities (due to vasodilatation)
- Mental status changes
- Decreased urine output
- Septic shock: Hyper- or hypothermia, tachypnea, tachycardia
- Neurogenic shock: Hypothermia, bradycardia
- Evidence of underlying infection (e.g., fever, sputum production, urinary symptoms) or CNS injury (e.g., history of trauma, focal neurologic deficits)

Diagnostic Evaluation

- Initial studies include CBC, electrolytes, renal function, lactate level (elevated in tissue hypoperfusion), PT/PTT, ABG to measures degree of acidosis (sepsis often has a respiratory alkalosis due to hyperventilation), and ECG
- Additional tests in cases of sepsis should include blood cultures, urinalysis with culture, CXR, CT of potentially infectious areas, cultures of infected lines or indwelling devices, DIC panel, and lumbar puncture
- Additional tests in cases of neurogenic shock include head CT and spinal X-ray/CT
- Swan-Ganz catheter placement may help identify the type of shock and guide management

	Cardiac Output	CVP/wedge pressure	SVR
Hypovolemic	↓	↓	↑
Neurogenic	↓	↓	↓
Septic	↑	↓	↓
Cardiogenic	↓	↑	↑

Treatment/Management

- Secure airway, establish two large-bore IVs (and possibly a central line), and administer supplemental O_2
- Administer large fluid volumes of normal saline or lactated Ringer's solution to compensate for the increased intravascular space
- Administer vasopressor drips (norepinephrine, dopamine, or phenylephrine)
- Neurogenic shock
  - Maintain C-spine protection
  - Atropine for symptomatic bradycardia
  - Methylprednisolone IV bolus and infusion in cases of blunt spinal cord injury
- Septic shock
  - Obtain blood, urine, and sputum cultures
  - Begin IV empiric antibiotics to cover likely pathogens based on the presenting clinical picture
  - Correct source of sepsis (e.g., bowel resection, cholecystectomy) or drain associated abscess

Prognosis/Complications

- Outcome depends on etiology and rapid restoration of adequate perfusion
- Continuously monitor for adequacy of resuscitation (e.g., stabilization of blood pressure, improvement of tachycardia, good perfusion on exam, resolution of acidosis, adequate urine output)
- Admit all patients with shock to an intensive care unit
- Persistent oxygen deprivation quickly causes irreversible cellular injury
- Sequelae include ARDS, cardiac ischemia, shock liver, DIC, neurologic damage, and acute renal failure due to ATN

81. Cardiogenic Shock

Etiology/Pathophysiology

- Cardiac output insufficient to meet metabolic demands, resulting in tissue hypoxia, despite *adequate* intravascular volume
- Hemodynamic criteria include hypotension, decreased cardiac output/index, and elevated pulmonary capillary occlusion pressure
- Three-quarters of patients diagnosed with cardiogenic shock have evidence of left ventricular dysfunction
- Intrinsic etiologies include MI (most common cause), valvular disease (e.g., acute mitral regurgitation), decompensated CHF, arrhythmias (e.g., due to electrolyte abnormalities), myocarditis, myocardial contusion, ventricular free wall or septal rupture, and dilated or hypertrophic cardiomyopathy
- Extrinsic etiologies (compressive, obstructive) include tension pneumothorax, pneumomediastinum, pericardial tamponade, mediastinal hematoma, diaphragmatic hernia, and positive pressure ventilation

Differential Dx

- Hypovolemic shock
  - Hemorrhage
  - Dehydration (e.g., diarrhea)
  - Extravascular fluid sequestration (third-spacing)
- Distributive shock
  - Septic shock
  - Neurogenic shock
- Hypoadrenal shock
- Anaphylaxis

Presentation/Signs & Symptoms

- Systolic BP <90 mmHg
- Pulse pressure (SBP-DBP) <20
- Cyanosis, ashen skin color, diaphoresis, mottled extremities
- Altered mental status
- Tachycardia
- Tachypnea
- Dyspnea
- Weak distal pulses
- Jugular venous distension
- Crackles in lungs
- Cardiac exam may reveal distant heart sounds, precordial heave, S_3, S_4, murmurs (e.g., mitral regurgitation, VSD)
- Oliguria

Diagnostic Evaluation

- ECG may reveal arrhythmias or acute myocardial infarction
- CXR often shows signs of CHF (e.g., vascular congestion, cephalization, Kerley B lines); may reveal underlying etiology (e.g., wide mediastinum in aortic dissection)
- Anion gap metabolic acidosis due to poor tissue perfusion
- Cardiac enzymes may be elevated in acute MI
- Echocardiogram (transthoracic and/or transesophageal) may be performed to assess ejection fraction, LV function, valvular function/regurgitation, pericardium for tamponade, free wall rupture, and ventricular septal defect
- Central venous catheterization reveals decreased cardiac output/index (<2.2 L/min/m^2), increased wedge pressure (>18 mmHg), increased systemic vascular resistance, and increased peripheral O_2 extraction
- Arterial line is recommended for blood pressure monitoring
- Cardiac catheterization is often diagnostic and may be therapeutic

Treatment/Management

- Airway control with intubation or CPAP as necessary
- Fluid resuscitation/blood transfusion to maximize cardiac filling and output
- IV inotrope administration: Dopamine (α- and β-agonist) if hypotensive to increase inotropy and vasoconstrict; dobutamine (β-agonist only) if normotensive to increase inotropy and vasodilate
- Avoid vasopressors (e.g., neosynephrine, norepinephrine) as they may improve blood pressure despite diminished tissue perfusion
- Correct arrhythmias immediately with cardioversion, external pacing, and medications
- PTCA is the preferred method for reperfusion in cases of cardiogenic shock following MI; thrombolytics are much less effective in shock states
- Correct electrolyte abnormalities as necessary
- Intra-aortic balloon pump may be used temporarily to ↓ afterload, thus improving perfusion and cardiac output

Prognosis/Complications

- Admit all patients to an ICU
- Overall mortality approaches 80%
- Mortality in the setting of an MI may exceed 80% with medical treatment alone, approaches 70% in patients who are administered fibrinolytics, and is 30% in patients treated with PTCA
- In general, the goal of initial therapy is to stabilize patients so that revascularization can be attempted
- Risk factors for the development of cardiogenic shock after an MI include increasing age, diabetes, decreased ejection fraction, large myocardial infarctions, female gender, multivessel disease, anterior wall MI, and history of a previous MI
- Shock most often occurs 6–7 hours after an acute MI

Head and Neck Disease

PHILLIP A. POLLICE, MD

82. Evaluation of a Neck Mass

Etiology/Pathophysiology

- Though nearly 100% of neck masses are benign, a mass occurring in a patient >30 must be considered a malignancy until proven otherwise
  - In pediatric and young adult populations (<30 years), inflammatory and congenital masses are far more common than neoplasms
  - In adult patients (>30 years), neoplasms are more common than inflammatory or congenital masses
  - Smoking, alcohol use, and history of head/neck radiation increase the likelihood of a malignant neoplasm
- Location of the neck mass is often helpful in narrowing the differential
  - Congenital cysts occur predictably based on type (e.g., thyroglossal cysts occur at the midline)
  - Location of upper aero-digestive tract malignant metastases are often predictable based upon primary site (e.g., tonsillar carcinoma metastases are often located in high jugular chain or level II of the neck)
- Duration of neck mass provides a clue to its etiology: 7 days suggests inflammatory lesion, 7 months suggests malignancy, 7 years suggests congenital lesion

Differential Dx

- Inflammatory mass
  - Lymphadenitis or abscess
  - Granulomatous process
- Congenital mass
  - Branchial cysts
  - Thyroglossal duct cyst
  - Dermoid
  - Lymphangioma
- Neoplastic mass
  - Local metastases (from upper aero-digestive tract)
  - Metastases from a distant site
  - Lymphoma
  - Thyroid carcinoma
  - Carotid body tumors
  - Glomus tumors
  - Schwannoma
  - Salivary gland tumors

Presentation/Signs & Symptoms

- Inflammatory masses often present with typical symptoms of infection (e.g., pain, erythema, tenderness, fluctuance, fever, leukocytosis)
- Congenital masses often present following an upper respiratory illness, with similar symptoms as inflammatory masses
  - May also present as asymptomatic, blottable neck masses
- Neoplastic masses usually present as asymptomatic and painless neck mass
  - Symptoms of malignant disease include weight loss, dysphagia/odynophagia, otalgia, change in voice, fetid odor, oral pain, and hemoptysis/hematemesis

Diagnostic Evaluation

- Complete head/neck exam is essential to identify potential primary tumor site
  - Note size and location of the mass
  - Note character of mass (e.g., firm, soft, blottable, pulsatile)
  - Office endoscopy should be used
- CT scan or MRI are the most helpful radiologic tests
- Ultrasound, arteriogram, and radionuclide scan are helpful in specific instances
- Fine needle aspiration will often make the diagnosis and guide management
  - "If you can feel a mass in the neck, put a needle in it"
- Surgical endoscopy with directed biopsy is used if a primary head/neck malignancy is suspected
- Open biopsy (incisional or excisional) is used as a last resort in cases that elude diagnosis despite the above workup

Treatment/Management

- Inflammatory neck masses require appropriate antibiotics, incision and drainage (e.g., for abscess), and/or excision
- Congenital neck masses may be excised or followed
- Neoplastic neck masses require excision or neck dissection
- Lymphoma requires excisional biopsy when possible

Prognosis/Complications

- Complications of neck surgery include bleeding, infection, chyle leak, cranial nerve injuries (V, VII, X, XI, XII), phrenic nerve injury, stroke, and brachial plexus injury

83. Surgical Thyroid Disease

Etiology/Pathophysiology

- Surgical thyroid disease includes thyroid cancer (see "Thyroid Neoplasms" entry), thyroid dysfunction states resulting in hyperthyroidism (including Graves' disease and toxic multinodular goiter), and diffuse thyroid enlargement (including diffuse multinodular goiter and chronic thyroiditis)
- Graves' disease (diffuse toxic non-nodular goiter): Auto-antibodies to the TSH receptor stimulate thyroid hormone production, resulting in hyperthyroidism
- Toxic multinodular goiter (Plummer's disease): Hyperfunctioning multiple nodules, resulting in hyperthyroidism
- Diffuse multinodular goiter: Non-functioning multiple nodules caused by adenomatous hyperplasia, resulting in a euthyroid state (most common cause of thyroid enlargement)
- Chronic thyroiditis: Hashimoto's disease and Riedel's (fibrous) thyroiditis
    - Hashimoto's disease: Autoimmune disorder that occurs mostly in women and results in enlargement of the thyroid gland with hypothyroidism
    - Riedel's (fibrous) thyroiditis: Thyroid gland is completely replaced by fibrous tissue, mimicking thyroid malignancy

Differential Dx

- Thyroid cancer
- Thyroid adenoma
- First-degree hyperthyroidism (e.g., Graves' disease, solitary adenoma, iodine ingestion, struma ovarii, toxic multinodular goiter, TSH-secreting pituitary adenoma, functioning thyroid cancer)
- Second-degree hyperthyroidism (e.g., pituitary adenoma, hCG-secreting tumor, gestational thyrotoxicosis, thyroid hormone resistance syndrome)
- Enlarged lymph node

Presentation/Signs & Symptoms

- Graves': Symptoms of hyperthyroidism (e.g., heat intolerance, sweating, irritability, weight loss, diarrhea, weakness, tremor, palpitations), proptosis, pretibial myxedema, exophthalmos
- Toxic multinodular goiter: Similar to Graves' disease, though patients may have a more subtle presentation
- Diffuse multinodular goiter: Usually asymptomatic; however, the enlarged thyroid may cause compressive symptoms of trachea or esophagus (e.g., pain, dysphagia, dyspnea)
- Hashimoto's disease: Hypothyroid state with a diffusely enlarged gland
- Riedel's thyroiditis: Rock-hard gland that may present with compressive symptoms

Diagnostic Evaluation

- Thyroid function tests and radionucleotide iodine scan are the primary means of diagnosis
- Graves' disease: Elevated thyroid hormones; diffuse uptake of iodine on radionucleotide iodine scan
- Toxic multinodular goiter: Elevated thyroid hormones; multiple distinct areas of uptake on radionucleotide scan
- Diffuse multinodular goiter: Normal thyroid function tests and radionucleotide scan
- Hashimoto's disease: Decreased thyroid hormones; poor uptake on radionucleotide scan; presence of antimicrosomal antibodies
- Riedel's thyroiditis: Normal thyroid function tests; poor uptake on radionucleotide scan; biopsy shows indeterminate fibrosis

Treatment/Management

- Graves' disease and toxic multinodular goiter
    - Radioactive iodine to ablate thyroid tissue is often definitive treatment (contraindicated in pregnancy)
    - Antithyroid drugs to interfere with thyroid hormone production (e.g., methimazole, propothiouracil)
    - Subtotal thyroidectomy is the treatment of choice if medical treatments are contraindicated or ineffective, or if suspect malignancy
- Diffuse multinodular goiter: Lifelong thyroid replacement therapy is the treatment of choice to suppress TSH stimulation of the thyroid; subtotal thyroidectomy is indicated if symptomatic or if medical therapy fails
- Hashimoto's disease: Thyroid replacement therapy; thyroidectomy is indicated if suspect malignancy or if medical therapy is ineffective
- Riedel's thyroiditis: Thyroidectomy to relieve compressive symptoms or if suspect malignancy

Prognosis/Complications

- Complications of thyroidectomy include thyroid storm, hemorrhage, compressive hematoma, hypothyroidism, hypoparathyroidism, and recurrent laryngeal nerve injury

84. Thyroid Neoplasms

Etiology/Pathophysiology

- Head and neck radiation is a strong risk factor for all thyroid cancers
- Papillary carcinoma of the thyroid (75% of cases)
  - Well-differentiated and easily curable
  - Females affected 3–4 times as often as males
  - Histology shows papillary fronds of epithelium, "Orphan Annie nuclei," and psammoma bodies
- Follicular carcinoma of the thyroid (10% of cases)
  - Common in iodine-deficient areas
  - Functions like normal thyroid tissue
  - Often curable
  - Females affected 3 times more frequently than males
  - Histology shows malignancy defined by capsular/vascular invasion
- Medullary carcinoma of the thyroid (10% of cases)
  - Cancer of calcitonin-producing C-cells
  - Associated with MEN-II syndromes
  - 80% are sporadic; 20% are familial
- Anaplastic carcinoma (5% of cases)
  - Poorly differentiated, aggressive tumors with poor prognosis
  - Histology shows undifferentiated spindle cells

Differential Dx

- Benign cysts
- Colloid nodules
- Adenoma
- Goiter
- Sarcoma
- Lymphoma
- Metastases
- Parathyroid cyst or cancer

Presentation/Signs & Symptoms

- Often presents as solitary nodule, though benign lesions make up the majority (85%) of thyroid nodules
- Papillary and follicular carcinoma are generally asymptomatic, but may present with change in voice, dysphagia/odynophagia, and adenopathy
- Medullary carcinoma often presents in patients with MEN-II syndromes or a strong family history of medullary carcinoma
- Anaplastic carcinoma presents as a rapidly growing neck mass; may have dysphagia, odynophagia, and/or hoarseness

Diagnostic Evaluation

- History and physical examination
- TSH level to rule out hyperthyroidism
- Elevated calcitonin in medullary carcinoma
- Ultrasound is used to detect nodules, distinguish between solid and cystic lesions, and aspirate cystic lesions
- Radioactive iodine (^{123}I) uptake scan reveals a "cold" nodule (i.e., no uptake of iodine)
  - Most malignant lesions are "cold" (i.e., no uptake of iodine)
  - However, only 15% of cold nodules are malignant
- Fine needle aspiration is the best diagnostic test (95% accuracy)
  - FNA cannot distinguish between follicular carcinoma and follicular adenoma because the diagnosis depends on evidence of invasion to adjacent structures)

Treatment/Management

- Thyroidectomy is the primary treatment for all thyroid cancers (except anaplastic), followed by postoperative radioactive ^{131}I ablation of remaining thyroid tissue and potential metastases
- Thyroid hormone replacement therapy
- Radiation and chemotherapy may be used palliatively for patients with advanced medullary cancer, but neither offer survival advantage
- Anaplastic cancers may be treated with radiation and radioactive ^{131}I, but neither is particularly effective
  - Tracheostomy and a feeding tube may be necessary

Prognosis/Complications

- Papillary carcinoma: >90% cure rate
- Follicular carcinoma: 70–80% cure rate
- Medullary carcinoma: 50–80% cure rate
- Anaplastic carcinoma: Dismal prognosis (uniformly fatal within 6 months)
- Metastases: Papillary carcinoma tends to spread via lymphatics to the cervical lymph nodes; follicular carcinoma tends to spread hematogenously to distant organs; medullary carcinoma spreads by both lymphatics and bloodstream
- Complications of surgery include recurrent laryngeal nerve or superior laryngeal nerve injuries, hypoparathyroidism, hematoma, seroma, infection, pneumothorax, thryotoxic storm, and tracheal or esophageal injury

85. Parathyroid Disease

Etiology/Pathophysiology

- Primary hyperparathyroidism is caused by a parathyroid adenoma (90% of cases), parathyroid hyperplasia, or parathyroid carcinoma
- Secondary hyperparathyroidism is caused by overstimulation of the parathyroid glands due to decreased serum calcium, usually secondary to chronic renal failure (parathyroid glands are normal)
- Parathyroid hormone increases blood calcium by stimulating breakdown of bone, increasing absorption from the gut, and decreasing renal excretion

Differential Dx

- Other causes of hypercalcemia (e.g., pseudohyperparathyroidism due to ectopic PTH), hyperthyroidism, malignancies, immobilization (e.g., Paget's disease), sarcoidosis, granulomatous disease (e.g., tuberculosis), excess vitamins A or D, thiazide diuretics, milk-alkali syndrome, familial hypocalciuric hypercalcemia, lithium use
- MEN-I syndrome
- MEN-IIa syndrome

Presentation/Signs & Symptoms

- Most cases are relatively asymptomatic; fatigue and other non-specific symptoms present
- "Stones, bones, abdominal groans, and psychic overtones" is the classic presentation of hypercalcemia; however, these are not common in clinical practice
    - *Stones*: Renal stones in 50%
    - *Bones* (osteitis fibrosa cystica): Bone pain, fractures, osteoporosis
    - *Groans*: Abdominal pain, nausea/vomiting, constipation, anorexia, PUD, pancreatitis
    - *Psychic overtones*: Psychosis, depression, fatigue, anxiety

Diagnostic Evaluation

- Serum calcium >10.5 mg/dL with elevated parathyroid hormone is diagnostic of primary hyperparathyroidism
- Markedly elevated serum calcium levels or a hypercalcemic crisis may suggest parathyroid carcinoma
- Ultrasound or CT of parathyroids may show an enlarged gland
- Sestamibi nuclear scan will highlight abnormal parathyroid gland(s)
- Selective venous sampling for parathyroid hormone levels may be indicated

Treatment/Management

- Parathyroidectomy is the treatment of choice
    - Adenomas require removal and verify that other parathyroid glands are normal by biopsy or inspection
    - Hyperplasia requires removal of 3½ glands
    - Carcinoma requires resection of parathyroid gland, ipsilateral thyroid gland, and any affected lymph nodes
- Severe hypercalcemia (calcium >13 mg/dL or symptoms) requires immediate intervention
    - IV rehydration with large volumes of normal saline
    - Loop diuretics to prevent volume overload and augment renal Ca^+ excretion

Prognosis/Complications

- Risks of parathyroid surgery include post-operative hypocalcemia (e.g., tetany, paresthesias, seizures), loss of airway, bleeding, hematoma, hoarseness, and recurrent laryngeal nerve damage

86. Sinusitis

Etiology/Pathophysiology

- Sinuses include maxillary, frontal, anterior and posterior ethmoids, and sphenoid
- Function of the sinuses is voice resonance, humidification of inspired air, and to decrease the weight of the skull
- Sinus function requires normal nasal secretions, ostial patency, and ciliary function
- Sinusitis results from any condition that disturbs normal physiology or anatomy (e.g., URI, nasal edema, nasal packing or intubation, nasal polyps, foreign bodies, ciliary dyskinesias)
- Acute sinusitis is usually due to viruses and bacteria (*S. pneumoniae, S. aureus, H. influenza,* group A *Streptococcus, Moraxella*)
- Chronic sinusitis may be due to the above organisms plus anaerobic bacteria, *Staphylococcus, Streptococcus, Pseudomonas,* fungi (e.g., Aspergillosis), or allergies
- Nosocomial sinusitis may be due to the above pathogens, methicillin-resistant *S. aureus* (MRSA), and vancomycin-resistant *enterococcus* (VRE)

Differential Dx

- Allergic rhinitis
- Non-allergic rhinitis
- Neoplasms (benign and malignant)
- Septal deformities
- Nasal polyposis
- Inverted papillomas
- Mucoceles
- Autoimmune diseases (e.g., Wegener's granulomatosis, sarcoidosis)

Presentation/Signs & Symptoms

- Purulent nasal drainage
- Nasal obstruction
- Pressure and pain (facial, nasal, retro-orbital)
- Headache
- Tenderness over the affected sinus
- Fever, lethargy, and malaise may be present

Diagnostic Evaluation

- History and physical examination
- Blood work is usually not helpful
- CT scan is the gold standard for diagnosis
    - Axial and coronal images will show air-fluid levels, opacification, or mucosal thickening
    - Mucosal thickening is more indicative of chronic disease
- MRI may be used but often exaggerates the degree of sinusitis
- Plain sinus X-rays are rarely helpful
- Cultures may be obtained by directed middle meatus and/or antral tap, especially for refractory cases

Treatment/Management

- Antibiotics may include penicillin, amoxicillin plus clavulanic acid, second or third generation cephalosporins, macrolides, and fluoroquinolones
    - Newer antibiotics are on the horizon (e.g., ketolides)
    - Steroids and decongestants (systemic and topical) are often helpful
    - Acute sinusitis is generally treated for 10–14 days; chronic sinusitis is often treated for 30 days or longer
    - Endoscopic sinus surgery is reserved for refractory chronic sinusitis to establish ostial patency

Prognosis/Complications

- Acute sinusitis is almost always curable if recognized and treated appropriately
- Chronic sinusitis may persist despite treatment
- Complications include orbital cellulitis or abscess, meningitis or epidural abscess, cranial nerve involvement (CN II, III, IV, V, VI), and brain abscess

87. Epistaxis

Etiology/Pathophysiology

- Bleeding from the nose may be anterior (through nares) or posterior (through nasopharynx and/or oropharynx)
- Anterior epistaxis (90% of nosebleeds) is generally a benign process that quickly resolves with therapy
    - Most commonly originates in Kiesselbach's plexus of vessels in the anterior nasal septum
- Posterior epistaxis is a much more serious bleed that originates in the large posterior nasal vessels and is more difficult to control—may result in significant blood loss, hypotension, or airway compromise
    - Often associated with hypertension, atherosclerosis, and older age
- Epistaxis occurs more frequently during the dry winter months, in dry heat, or with abrupt temperature changes

Differential Dx

- Trauma
- Iatrogenic (e.g., nasal intubations, nasal cannula oxygen)
- Infections
- Septal deformities (due to abnormal air currents and dryness)
- Tumors
- Osler-Weber-Rendu syndrome
- Coagulopathies (blood dyscrasias, anticoagulant medications)

Presentation/Signs & Symptoms

- Anterior epistaxis
    - Unilateral bleeding
    - Minimal or no blood in the posterior pharynx
    - Dried clots
    - Nasal crusting
    - Visible bleeding site
- Posterior epistaxis
    - Bilateral bleeding
    - Blood or clots in the oropharynx
    - No visible anterior lesions
    - Fails to resolve with anterior packing

Diagnostic Evaluation

- History and physical examination
    - Visualize interior of the nose with a headlamp, rhinoscopy, and/or nasal endoscopy
- CBC and PT/PTT may be ordered in cases of anterior epistaxis if a coagulopathy is suspected
- CBC, blood type and screen, and PT/PTT in significant cases of posterior epistaxis
- Consider CT of the head and facial bones if epistaxis is the result of trauma or if suspect neoplasm
- Arteriogram in severe cases

Treatment/Management

- Anterior epistaxis
    - Maintain direct pressure for at least 10 minutes
    - Intranasal vasoconstrictors (e.g., phenylephrine)
    - Cauterization (silver nitrate or electrocautery) may be attempted if the site of bleeding is identified
    - Nasal packing should be attempted if cautery fails
    - Antibiotics covering *Staphylococcus* may be given after packing to prevent toxic shock syndrome
    - Endoscopically guided cautery may be necessary
    - Septoplasty may be indicated for recurrent anterior epistaxis secondary to septal deviation
- Posterior epistaxis
    - Vasoconstrictors and anesthetics may be useful
    - Nasal packing with balloon tamponade
    - Definitive care may require embolization of the internal maxillary and facial arteries or endoscopic sphenopalatine ligation

Prognosis/Complications

- Anterior epistaxis is often recurrent and self-limited
- Posterior epistaxis is often severe, persistent, and may be life-threatening
- When bleeding is controlled, prognosis is generally good
- Cessation of bleeding often takes 3–5 days of packing; follow-up is necessary
- Complications include infection (e.g., sinusitis) and sequelae of bleeding (e.g., low hematocrit, hypotension, poor perfusion)

88. Oral Cavity Neoplasms

Etiology/Pathophysiology

- Oral cavity malignancies comprise 40% of all head and neck malignancies
- The oral cavity begins at the skin-vermillion border of the lips to the circumvellate papillae of tongue
  - Includes hard palate and gingiva to hard/soft palate junction
  - Includes anterior two-thirds of tongue and floor of mouth
  - Includes alveolar surfaces of mandible and maxilla
- Risk factors for malignancy include tobacco use (smoking and chewing tobacco), alcohol abuse, reverse smoking, and betel-nut chewing (Asia)
- 95% of patients are >40 years (average 60 years)
- 95% of oral cavity malignancies are squamous cell carcinoma
- Oral cavity lesions, irritations, masses, or ill-fitting dentures lasting more than 2 weeks require workup and biopsy

Differential Dx

- Squamous cell carcinoma
- Adenoid cystic carcinoma
- Adenocarcinoma
- Mucoepidermoid carcinoma
- Sarcoma
- Melanoma
- Lymphoma
- Premalignant lesions (e.g., leukoplakia, erythroplakia)
- Benign tumors (e.g., sialometaplasia, neuroma, granular cell myoblastoma)

Presentation/Signs & Symptoms

- Painful oral mass
- Otalgia (earache)
- Oral pain
- Odynophagia and dysphagia
- Bleeding
- Unexpected loss or loosening of teeth
- Trismus
- Weight loss
- Oral fetor

Diagnostic Evaluation

- Complete head and neck examination
- Direct oral biopsy of suspicious masses, ulcers, or lesions
- CT scan or MRI of neck (with contrast)
- Panendoscopy (direct laryngoscopy, esophagoscopy, and bronchoscopy) to rule out synchronous tumors
- Staging (TNM classification)
  - T1: Tumor 2 cm or less; T2: Tumor 2–4 cm; T3: Tumor >4 cm; T4: Tumor invades bone, deep tongue muscle, and skin
  - N0: No regional lymph node (LN) metastases; N1: Single regional LN, 3 cm or less; N2a: Single ipsilateral LN, >3 —6 cm; N2b: Multiple ipsilateral LN, but none >6 cm; N2c: Bilateral or contralateral LN, but none >6 cm; N3: LN metastases >6 cm
  - Mx: Unknown metastases; M0: No metastases; M1: Known metastases

Treatment/Management

- Surgical resection of primary tumor
  - Partial to complete glossectomy
  - Partial palatectomy to maxillectomy
  - Composite resection with extirpation of bone and soft tissue en bloc
- Reconstruction of primary site may include primary closure, split thickness skin grafting, myocutaneous flaps, and free tissue transfer
- Neck dissection is indicated for clinical disease (i.e., palpable nodes) or >20% probability of occult nodal metastasis (T2, T3, or T4 lesions)
- Radiation and chemotherapy postoperatively

Prognosis/Complications

- Prognosis varies with site of malignancy and degree of treatment
- Earlier diagnosis and earlier stage has better prognosis
- Complications vary with extent of surgery and extent of disease, may include articulation difficulty, swallowing difficulty, and cranial nerve deficits
- Complications of neck dissections include bleeding, infection, chyle (lymph) leak, cranial nerve injury (V, VII, X, XI, XII), phrenic nerve injury, stroke, and brachial plexus injury

89. Salivary Gland Neoplasms

Etiology/Pathophysiology

- The major salivary glands include pairs of parotid, submandibular, and sublingual glands
- The minor salivary glands include 600–1000 glands throughout the upper aerodigestive tract
- History of radiation exposure and occupational exposure to woods have been associated with salivary gland neoplasms
- Parotid glands accounts for 80% of salivary gland neoplasms (80% benign; 20% malignant)
- Submandibular glands account for 10–15% of salivary gland neoplasms (50% benign; 50% malignant)
- Sublingual and minor salivary glands account for 5–10% of salivary gland neoplasms (40% benign; 60% malignant)
- Pleomorphic adenoma is the most common type of benign salivary gland neoplasm; Warthin's tumor (papillary cystadenoma lymphomatosum) is the second most common benign neoplasm
- Mucoepidemoid carcinoma is the most common malignant neoplasm of the salivary glands; adenoid cystic carcinoma is the second most common

Differential Dx

- Infectious parotitis
- Sialoadenitis
- Autoimmune parotitis (e.g., Sjogren's syndrome, Wegener's granulomatosis)
- Metastases
- Lymphoma
- Benign neoplasms (e.g., pleomorphic adenoma, Warthin's tumor, monomorphic adenoma, sebaceous adenoma)
- Malignant neoplasms (e.g., mucoepidermoid, adenoid cystic, ex-pleomorphic, acinous, adenocarcinoma, squamous cell)

Presentation/Signs & Symptoms

- Painless, slowly growing mass in the region of the parotid, submandibular, sublingual, or minor salivary glands
- Signs of malignancy include fixation, local invasion, facial nerve involvement (paralysis), and other cranial nerve involvement

Diagnostic Evaluation

- History and physical examination
- Fine needle aspiration
- CT scan or MRI are used in some cases
- Parotidectomy is only appropriate surgical biopsy— incisional biopsy is *contraindicated*
- Staging (TNM system)
  - T1: Tumor 2 cm or less; T2: Tumor 2–4 cm; T3: Tumor 4–6 cm; T4: Tumor >6 cm
  - N0: No regional lymph node (LN) metastases; N1: Single regional LN, 3 cm or less; N2a: Single ipsilateral LN, >3 —6 cm; N2b: Multiple ipsilateral LN, but none >6 cm; N2c: Bilateral or contralateral LN, but none >6 cm; N3: LN metastases >6 cm
  - Mx: Unknown metastases; M0: No metastases; M1: Known metastases

Treatment/Management

- Superficial parotidectomy with identification and preservation or facial nerve is indicated for benign tumors of the superficial lobe and malignancies without cranial nerve VII involvement
- Radical parotidectomy with removal of all parotid tissue and sacrifice of the facial nerve is reserved for aggressive malignancies, cranial nerve VII involvement, recurrent benign disease that has failed other treatments (e.g., recurrent pleomorphic adenoma)
- Neck dissections for clinically positive disease (i.e., palpable nodes)
- Adjuvant radiation and chemotherapy for unresectable disease or postoperatively in aggressive malignancies

Prognosis/Complications

- Parotidectomy is curative for benign tumors
- High grade malignant tumors (e.g., mucoepidermoid, squamous cell, and adenocarcinomas) have a poor prognosis
- Complications of parotid surgery include facial nerve injury (paralysis), infection, bleeding, hematoma, sialocele and seroma, Frey's sydrome (gustatory sweating), auricular hypoesthesia (greater auricular nerve sacrifice), and cosmetic deformity

90. Laryngeal Neoplasms

Etiology/Pathophysiology

- Laryngeal cancer accounts for 25% of all head and neck malignancies
- Anatomy
  - Supraglottis: Tip of epiglottis to apices of ventricles (includes epiglottis, false vocal folds, arytenoids, and aryepiglottic folds)
  - Glottis: At level of the true vocal folds
  - Subglottis: 5 mm inferior to the true vocal folds to the inferior border of the cricoid cartilage (includes subglottic trachea)
- Laryngeal functions include respiration, airway protection during swallowing, and phonation
  - Phonation may be sacrificed for surgical extirpation, but the functions of respiration and swallowing must be restored
- Risk factors for laryngeal malignancies include tobacco use, alcohol abuse, and GERD
- The true vocal fold is the origin of laryngeal cancer in up to 75% of cases
- Lymph node metastases tend to occur in advanced stage disease secondary to the relative paucity of lymphatics within larynx

Differential Dx

- Squamous cell carcinoma (>95% of laryngeal malignancies)
- Verrucous carcinoma
- Sarcoma
- Chondroma
- Minor salivary gland carcinoma
- Granulomatous diseases (e.g., tuberculosis, sarcoidosis, Wegener's granulomatosis)
- Benign tumors (e.g., granular cell tumors, papillomas)
- Benign lesions (e.g., nodules, cysts, granulomas)

Presentation/Signs & Symptoms

- Hoarseness is the cardinal symptom of laryngeal cancer (persistent hoarseness longer than 2 weeks requires evaluation)
- Dysphagia (difficulty swallowing)
- Odynophagia (painful swallowing)
- Sense of fullness in throat
- Otalgia (ear pain)
- Hemoptysis
- Stridor and/or dyspnea
- Weight loss

Diagnostic Evaluation

- Full head and neck exam
- Laryngoscopy (mirror, flexible fiberoptic, video)
- CT scan or MRI of neck (with contrast)
- Panendoscopy (direct laryngoscopy, esophagoscopy, and bronchoscopy) with directed biopsies
- Staging (TNM classification)
  - T1a: Tumor limited to one vocal fold
  - T1b: Tumor involving both vocal folds
  - T2: Tumor extends to supra- or subglottis and/or vocal fold motion impairment
  - T3: Tumor limited to larynx with vocal fold fixation
  - T4: Tumor invading thyroid cartilage or outside larynx to oropharynx, hypopharynx, soft tissues of neck

Treatment/Management

- Surgical resection of primary laryngeal tumor may be accomplished by endoscopic resection, partial laryngectomy, supracricoid laryngectomy, or total laryngectomy with voice restoration surgery
- Primary radiation therapy is indicated for early tumors (T1, T2)
- Organ preservation protocols (chemotherapy, radiation) may be used as primary treatment for T1, T2, and T3 tumors
- Neck dissection if a palpable node is felt or advanced primary disease (T3, T4)
- Radiation and chemotherapy postoperatively in advanced disease

Prognosis/Complications

- Prognosis varies with extent of disease
  - T1 cancer: 90% cure rate
  - T2 cancer: 80% cure rate
  - T3 and T4 cancers: 50–60% cure rate
- Complications of surgery include wound infection, pharyngocutaneous fistula, hypothyroidism, pharyngeal stenosis, and stomal stenosis
- Complications of radiation and chemotherapy include hematologic complications, mucositis, dryness, dysphagia, hypothyroidism, and osteoradionecrosis

91. Obstructive Sleep Apnea

Etiology/Pathophysiology

- A syndrome of repetitive periods of apnea (>10 seconds without air flow) or hypopnea during sleep, resulting in desaturations and poor sleep
- Sleep apnea may be obstructive, central, or mixed (however, symptoms are similar regardless of type)
  - Central sleep apnea occurs due to absent signals to breathe from the CNS respiratory center, resulting in apnea without a respiratory effort
  - Obstructive sleep apnea (OSA) occurs when upper airway soft tissue impedes airflow
- OSA tends to worsen with age and weight gain (obesity is a major factor)
  - Aging results in loss of upper airway turgor
  - Weight gain narrows the upper airway and promotes airway collapse
  - Risk factors for OSA include narrow airways (obesity, macroglossia), alcohol, sedatives, URI, hypothyroidism, smoking, vocal cord dysfunction, and bulbar disease
  - Occurs in 4% of males and 2% of females
- OSA is strongly linked to significant morbidity and mortality due to sudden nocturnal death (likely related to arrhythmias), pulmonary hypertension and resulting cor pulmonale, heart failure, pulmonary edema, hypertension, stroke, and accidents (industrial, automobile) due to hypersomnolence

Differential Dx

- Primary snoring without apnea
- Sleep deprivation
- Narcolepsy
- Nocturnal myoclonus
- Hypothyroidism
- Central sleep apnea
- Obstructive neoplasms
- Vocal fold paralysis (both unilateral and bilateral)
- Post-surgical obstructions
- Primary alveolar hypoventilation ("Ondine's curse")
- Obesity-Hypoventilation syndrome (Pickwickian syndrome)

Presentation/Signs & Symptoms

- Snoring is cardinal symptom
- Daytime somnolence (e.g., falling asleep at the wheel or on the couch)
- Nighttime arousals
- Apnea during sleep
- Weight gain
- Oropharyngeal exam may reveal tonsillar hypertrophy, large base of tongue, long soft palate, narrow oropharyngeal airway, micrognathia, or retrognathia
- Nasal obstruction
- The patient's bed partner may provide the most useful information

Diagnostic Evaluation

- Workup is appropriate when nocturnal problems are contributing to secondary daytime behavioral and physiologic problems
- History and physical exam, including nasal and nasopharyngeal examination
- Fiberoptic endoscopy (in office)
- Overnight pulse oximetry is a useful screening test
- Sleep studies (polysomnography and multiple sleep latency testing) can provide a definitive diagnosis
- Radiography may include cephalograms (cephalometrics), CT scan and MRI, and somnofluoroscopy
- Thyroid function tests to rule out hypothyroidism

Treatment/Management

- Avoid alcohol and sedatives in patients with increased upper airway muscle tone
- For patients with narrowed upper airway lumen size, weight reduction may be curative
- Nighttime nasal CPAP (continuous positive airway pressure) is the treatment of choice
- Oral dental prosthesis may be useful
- Tonsillectomy/uvulopalatopharyngoplasty is the procedure of choice in selected patients who have failed the above therapies
  - Other procedures may include genioglossus advancement, hyoid suspension, and maxillary or mandibular advancement
- Tracheostomy may be necessary to bypass the obstruction in patients with life-threatening complications and failure of other therapies

Prognosis/Complications

- Sleep apnea *does* cause increased mortality
- Sleep apnea syndrome is one of the leading causes of daytime sleepiness
- Prognosis is good when properly identified and treated
- CPAP is nearly 100% effective when worn properly; however, may be uncomfortable
- Complications of advanced disease include hypertension, arrhythmias and sudden death, pulmonary hypertension and cor pulmonale, left heart failure, and stroke

92. Vocal Fold Paralysis

Etiology/Pathophysiology

- Neural anatomy of the larynx
  - Recurrent laryngeal nerve is a branch of cranial nerve X (vagus nerve): Motor innervation to the intrinsic muscles of the larynx (abduction, adduction, phonation); sensory innervation to the trachea and subglottis
  - Superior laryngeal nerve is also a branch of the vagus nerve: Motor innervation to the cricothyroid muscle (lengthening, shortening, pitch changes); sensory innervation to the larynx and pharynx
- Functions of the larynx include respiration, airway protection during swallowing, and phonation
- Unilateral vocal fold paralysis is caused by unilateral recurrent laryngeal nerve dysfunction, and the vocal fold is usually fixed in a paramedian position
- Bilateral vocal fold paralysis is caused by bilateral recurrent laryngeal nerve dysfunction, and the vocal folds are fixed in the midline position
- Superior laryngeal nerve paralysis results in sensory dysfunction of the glottis and supraglottis and motor dysfunction of the cricothyroid

Differential Dx

- Infection (usually viral)
- Neurodegenerative processes
- Trauma
- Idiopathic
- Neoplasms (benign and malignant) of the skull base, lung, esophagus, thyroid, larynx, or nerves
- Surgery of the skull base, thoracic, carotid, thyroid, cardiac, esophageal, laryngeal, cervical spine

Presentation/Signs & Symptoms

- Unilateral vocal fold paralysis
  - Hoarseness
  - Aspiration (e.g., cough, pneumonia)
  - Airway is intact
- Bilateral vocal fold paralysis
  - Airway obstruction
  - Stridor
  - Voice is relatively normal
- Superior laryngeal nerve paralysis
  - Voice is often normal
  - Unable to change pitch (e.g., cannot sing)
  - Aspiration (e.g., cough, pneumonia)

Diagnostic Evaluation

- History and physical examination
- Diagnostic laryngoscopy via flexible fiberoptic, rigid videolaryngoscopy, mirror examination, or direct surgical examination (less useful)
- Laryngeal EMG studies
- CT scan and MRI (from skull base to thoracic inlet) are used to identify potential etiologies

Treatment/Management

- Unilateral vocal fold paralysis: Objective of treatment is to medialize the paralyzed vocal fold
  - Vocal fold injections of gelfoam, fat, or collagen; Teflon for advanced cases
  - Medialization thyroplasty or type I thyroplasty (silastic, cartilage, hydroxylapatite, Goretex)
  - Arytenoid adduction
  - Re-innervation procedures
- Bilateral vocal fold paralysis: Objective of treatment is to establish an airway and maintain voice, if possible
  - Tracheostomy
  - Laser cordotomy or cordectomy
  - Arytenoidectomy or arytenoidopexy

Prognosis/Complications

- Unilateral vocal fold paralysis may result in hoarseness and aspiration
- Bilateral vocal fold paralysis may result in stridor, reasonable voice, and airway obstruction; the airway is established at the expense of voice

Urology

RALPH J. MILLER, JR., MD, FACS
JOHN C. LYNE, MD

93. Urology Anatomy, Facts, and Pearls

- The entire urinary tract from the collecting system of the kidney to the distal urethra is lined by transitional epithelium, with the distal female urethra, and the male anterior urethra lined by squamous epithelium
- The adrenals, kidneys, and ureters are retroperitoneal
- The posterior wall of the bladder lies in the retroperitoneum; the dome of the bladder is intraperitoneal; the anterior wall of the bladder lies in the anterior pre-peritoneal space (space of Retzius)
- The ureters leave the renal pelvis behind the great renal vessels and descend in a medial position until they flare out laterally as they enter the bony pelvis; they then descend medially over the distal common iliac vein and artery before entering the base of the bladder; the narrowest points of the ureters (hence the places where stones become impacted) are the ureteropelvic junction, the point over the pelvic vessels, and the ureterovesical junction
- The female urethra is about 4 cm long and extends from the bladder neck, through the perineum and external sphincter, and ends at the meatus situated on the anterior vaginal wall
- The male urethra is divided into three distinct regions: The posterior urethra extends from the bladder neck through the prostate to the external sphincter; the bulbar urethra widens between the proximal corpora cavernosa bodies; the penile urethera extends distally
- The prostate is a walnut-shaped gland situated between the bladder and external sphincter, enveloped in a fused fascial coating known as Denonvilliers fascia; the prostate is fixed to the underside of the pubic symphysis (in cases of pelvic trauma, this fixation can result in disruption of the posterior urethra)
- The testes originates in the retroperitoneum and takes with them a covering of peritoneum as they descend through the inguinal canal shortly before birth to rest within the scrotum; the venous drainage of the testis is via the gonadal vein, which enters the inferior vena cava on the right and the renal vein on the left; incompetence of the valves of the left vein can result in a varicocele, affecting 15% of the male population

94. Pyelonephritis

Etiology/Pathophysiology

- Acute pyelonephritis is a bacterial infection of the renal parenchyma or collecting system
- Chronic pyelonephritis (characterized by scarring and parenchymal loss) may follow multiple infections, chronic obstruction, and vesicoureteral reflux
- Most cases of upper urinary tract infections are due to ascending bacteria from the lower urinary tract; however, hematogenous spread may play a role in some cases (e.g., renal parenchymal abscess in an IV drug user)
- Emphysematous pyelonephritis is a severe, life-threatening, necrotizing infection caused by gas forming organisms

Differential Dx

- Lower urinary tract infection
- Urolithiasis
- Pelvic inflammatory disease
- Appendicitis
- Diverticulitis
- Cholecystitis
- Retroperitoneal hemorrhage
- Pneumonia

Presentation/Signs & Symptoms

- Flank pain
- Fever/chills
- Nausea/vomiting
- Lower urinary tract symptoms (e.g., dysuria, frequency, urgency, sense of incomplete voiding)
- CVA tenderness
- Severe pyelonephritis may present as a toxic or septic condition (e.g., mental status changes, hypotension)

Diagnostic Evaluation

- A history of recurrent UTIs, diabetes, stones, recent procedures, or IV drug use may be present
- Urinalysis will reveal pyuria and bacteriuria
- Urine and blood cultures should be taken prior to beginning antibiotic therapy
- CBC with differential cell counts
- Renal ultrasound may be necessary to rule out an obstruction or a large abscess
- In severe infections or patients not responding to antibiotics, a CT scan or intravenous pyelogram may be indicated to assess for gas in the parenchyma or abscess formation

Treatment/Management

- Initiate IV antibiotics as soon as cultures are taken
  - Begin empiric treatment with ampicillin and an aminoglycoside until definitive organism is identified
  - In acute pyelonephritis, IV antibiotics are continued for 2–6 days, until fever decreases
  - Oral therapy is commenced once fever declines and is continued for at least 14 days
- Vigorous IV hydration for patients with sepsis
- Percutaneous drainage of associated abscesses
- Retrograde stent placement or percutaneous nephrostomy is indicated for upper urinary tract obstruction and emphysematous pyelonephritis
- Nephrectomy may be necessary in severe emphysematous pyelonephritis

Prognosis/Complications

- Renal abscess or perinephric abscess may result as a complication of an upper tract infection
- Chronic pyelonephritis may result in shrunken, scarred kidneys and ensuing renal insufficiency and hypertension

95. Renal Cell Carcinoma

Etiology/Pathophysiology

- 90% of solid renal masses are renal cell carcinomas
  - Note that most solid renal masses are malignant and most cystic lesions are benign
- Peak incidence during age 40–60, with a male predominance
- Risk factors include smoking, heavy metal exposure (cadmium), female obesity, and familial disorders (e.g., von Hippel Landau disease, hereditary renal papillary carcinoma)
- Arises from the proximal convoluted tubule
- Histologic varieties include clear cell (>80% of cases), chromophobe, and papillary
- Spreads to nodes, lungs, liver, bone, thyroid, and brain

Differential Dx

- Wilms' tumor (most common solid tumor of childhood)
- Renal cysts (simple cyst, complex cyst, acquired cystic disease)
- Inherited cystic disease (polycystic kidney disease, von Hippel Lindau)
- Angiomyolipoma
- Hydronephrosis
- Neuroblastoma
- Transitional cell carcinoma of the renal pelvis
- Lymphoma
- Sarcoma (generally leiomyosarcoma)

Presentation/Signs & Symptoms

- Patients are usually asymptomatic until the carcinoma becomes quite large
- Flank pain
- Hematuria
- Palpable mass
- Weight loss/cachexia
- Hypertension
- Hypercalcemia

Diagnostic Evaluation

- Most cases are discovered incidentally on abdominal imaging studies
- CT with or without contrast is the test of choice to distinguish renal cell carcinoma from benign cysts
  - CT also allows assessment of local tumor advancement (through the renal capsule to Gerota's fascia), regional nodes, liver metastases, and contralateral renal function
- MRI is indicated in cases where renal vein and IVC involvement are suspected and in patients where CT contrast is contraindicated (e.g., renal failure, dye allergy)
- Renal arteriography to evaluate the arterial anatomy if partial nephrectomy is being contemplated
- Metastatic workup should include a chest X-ray, LFTs, bone scan, and head CT
- Elevated hemoglobin may be present
- Urine cytology is rarely helpful

Treatment/Management

- Surgical resection is the treatment of choice
  - Indicated in localized disease or in advanced symptomatic cases
  - Smaller (<4 cm) tumors can be excised or treated with laparoscopic or percutaneous cryoablation or radiofrequency ablation
  - Radical nephrectomy (including resection of adrenal gland, Gerota's fascia, and regional lymph nodes) is performed for larger or advanced tumors; most cases can be performed laparoscopically
- Radiation is used for palliation of bony metastases
- The only proven therapy for metastatic disease is immunotherapy (IL-2 or interferon), which induces a response in 20% of patients

Prognosis/Complications

- Increased risk of metastasis once the tumor exceeds 5 cm
- Staging
  - T1: <7 cm within kidney
  - T2: >7 cm within kidney
  - T3: Through capsule, into adrenal gland, into renal vein, or into IVC
  - T4: Involvement beyond Gerota's fascia (fascial envelope of the kidney) into adjacent structures
- Survival is >90% for T1, 50–75% for T3, and very poor for T4

96. Benign Prostatic Hyperplasia

Etiology/Pathophysiology

- The exact cause of benign prostatic hyperplasia (BPH) is unknown, but it is related to aging and the effects of testosterone on the balance between cell growth and cell death in the prostate
- The prostate gland generally begins to enlarge in the fifth decade of life
- As the prostate gland enlarges, lower urinary tract symptoms occur, likely caused by impingement of the enlarged gland on the urethra
  - Fixed mechanical outflow obstruction
  - Dynamic outflow obstruction
  - Secondary bladder irritability

Differential Dx

- Urethral stricture
- Bladder cancer
- Bladder calculus
- Infection (e.g., prostatitis, cystitis)
- Neurogenic bladder
- Prostate cancer

Presentation/Signs & Symptoms

- Obstructive symptoms predominate
  - Weak stream
  - Hesitancy
  - Intermittency
  - Sense of incomplete bladder emptying
  - Post-void dribbling
- Irritative symptoms are also common
  - Frequency
  - Urgency
  - Nocturia
- Urinary retention is an uncommon presentation
- Untreated BPH can present as renal failure with overflow incontinence

Diagnostic Evaluation

- History and physical exam will usually reveal obstructive symptoms; if only irritative symptoms are present, other diagnoses should be considered (e.g., infection, prostatitis, bladder cancer)
  - Digital rectal exam is indicated to evaluate the size, consistency, and presence of nodules in the prostate
  - Abdominal exam should evaluate for distension of the bladder
- Urinalysis should be done to rule out other conditions (e.g., pyuria in infections, hematuria in many other conditions)
- Measure PSA as a screening to rule out prostate cancer
- Electrolytes and BUN/creatinine are indicated to evaluate renal function in patients with urinary retention
- Upper urinary tract imaging (CT, ultrasound, or IVP) to evaluate for obstruction or other treatable conditions

Treatment/Management

- Treatment is based on the severity of symptoms; symptoms and degree of obstruction correlates poorly with size of prostate on exam
- Observation alone is generally sufficient for patients with mild symptoms; some patients opt for phytotherapy (e.g., saw palmetto)
- Patients with increasing symptoms may be started on a trial of an α-blocker or finasteride
- Patients with severe obstruction, urinary retention, or impairment of renal function generally require transurethral resection of the prostate (TURP); however, several minimally invasive therapies are now also available

Prognosis/Complications

- Prognosis is generally good whether managed medically or surgically
- Untreated BPH can lead to urinary tract infection, bladder calculi, renal failure, or urinary retention that persists in spite of relief of obstruction

97. Prostatitis

Etiology/Pathophysiology

- A bacterial infection or non-bacterial inflammation of the prostate
- May be acute or chronic
- The most common etiologic organisms are *E. coli, Klebsiella, Enterococcus, Staphylococcus* species, and *Candida*
- Infection often occurs via retrograde spread through the urethra
- May be associated with sexually transmitted diseases, such as gonorrhea or chlamydia

Differential Dx

- Cystitis/urethritis
- Chronic pelvic pain syndrome (prostatodynia)
- Bladder cancer
- Prostate cancer
- Calculous disease
- Benign prostatic hyperplasia
- Urinary retention
- Neurologic disease

Presentation/Signs & Symptoms

- Urinary frequency and urgency
- Dysuria
- Urinary retention
- Pain may occur in the perineum, low back, pelvis, testes, or supapubic area
- Pain with ejaculation
- Fever/chills
- Tender boggy prostate on physical exam

Diagnostic Evaluation

- Microscopic examination of prostatic fluid (expressed by prostatic massage) is generally diagnostic
  - Large numbers of WBCs will be present in patients with bacterial prostatitis
  - Avoid prostate massage if the prostate is very tender or if the patient is febrile, as bacteremia may occur
- Urinalysis will reveal pyuria in patients with bacterial prostatitis
- Urine culture may reveal the offending organism
- Prostatic fluid culture may be done in some cases
- PSA levels may be falsely elevated during acute prostatitis

Treatment/Management

- Administer oral antibiotics based on patient characteristics
  - Treat for gram-negative organisms in older populations (e.g., trimethoprim-sulfamethoxazole, fluoroquinolone)
  - Treat for sexually transmitted organisms in younger populations (e.g., tetracycline, fluoroquinolone)
  - Penicillins and cephalosporins have poor prostatic penetration and should be avoided
  - Initial therapy is typically 30–45 days; chronic prostatitis may require extended treatment
  - Febrile or toxic patients may require IV antibiotics
- Chronic cases may benefit from prostatic massage, herbal therapies, intraprostatic antibiotic injection, or transurethral resection of the prostate (TURP)

Prognosis/Complications

- Acute prostatitis has a high cure rate
- Chronic prostatitis can be aggravatingly recurrent or persistent
- Complications may include urinary retention, urosepsis, and prostatic abscess
- Screening for prostate cancer should be done in appropriate patients (e.g., age >50) once prostatitis has resolved

98. Prostate Cancer

Etiology/Pathophysiology

- Prostate cancer is the most common visceral malignancy in men
- Second leading cause of cancer death in men
- Factors associated with increased incidence include advancing age, high animal fat diet, Northern latitudes, African-American race in the U.S., and family history
- Possible preventative factors include a low fat diet, anti-oxidant vitamins, lycopene, selenium, and soy proteins
- The presence of testosterone is necessary but not sufficient for the development of prostate cancer
- Nearly 100% of cases are adenocarcinoma
- Metastasizes to lymph nodes and bone marrow

Differential Dx

- Benign prostatic nodule
- Benign prostatic hyperplasia
- Prostatitis
- Rectal mass
- Prostatic abscess
- Urinary tract infection

Presentation/Signs & Symptoms

- Most cases are asymptomatic and present only with an elevated PSA on screening
- Non-specific obstructive urinary symptoms may be present (e.g., frequency, weak stream, retention)
- Hematuria
- Hard prostate nodule may be palpated on digital rectal exam
- A small percentage of cases present with sequellae of metastatic disease, such as back pain (from vertebral metastases), renal failure (from ureteral obstruction), or weight loss

Diagnostic Evaluation

- Historically, most cases were discovered incidentally on rectal exam or on examination of the prostate tissue following a transurethral resection of the prostate
- Today, most cases are detected by prostate-specific antigen (PSA) screening
- Transrectal ultrasound of the prostate with prostate biopsy (ultrasound alone is not helpful)
- Depending on the PSA, tumor grade, and tumor stage, a metastatic evaluation may be warranted
  - Bone scan
  - CT of the abdomen and pelvis
  - Prostascint scan (antibodies tagged against prostate-specific membrane antigen)

Treatment/Management

- For localized disease, four potentially curative options are available: Prostatectomy, external beam radiation, internal radiation (brachytherapy), and cryosurgery
- Depending on patient age, health, and tumor status, "watchful waiting" (observation alone with no active treatment) may be acceptable
- Gonadotropin releasing hormone (GnRH) agonists (e.g., leuprolide) are used as androgen deprivation therapy to reduce circulating testosterone
  - May be used as adjuvant or primary therapy for localized disease
  - Usually used as primary therapy for advanced disease
- Chemotherapy for prostate cancer is an area under active development; though chemotherapy has been ineffective in the past, some signs of success are emerging

Prognosis/Complications

- Prognosis is excellent with early diagnosis
- For localized disease, there is 85% 10-year survival, even with no treatment
- Cure rates with surgery for early stage lesions exceed 90%
- Most complications result from metastatic spread or locally advanced neoplasm (e.g., weight loss, anemia, pathologic fractures, renal failure, bladder outlet obstruction, hematuria)
- Complications of treatment include post-operative infection, erectile dysfunction, incontinence, retrograde ejaculation, and radiation proctitis
- Average life expectancy for patients with metastatic disease is 2–5 years

99. Bladder Cancer

Etiology/Pathophysiology

- Transitional cell carcinoma accounts for >90% of cases
  - Neoplasm arises from the transitional epithelium that lines the renal collecting system (calyces and pelvis), ureters, bladder, and proximal urethra
  - Risk factors include cigarette smoking, exposure to various chemicals (e.g., azo and aniline dyes), and benzene-containing compounds
  - Bladder is most common site of transitional cell carcinomas
- Squamous cell and adenocarcinoma are much less common
- Metastases occur to the regional lymph nodes, liver, lungs, bone, and brain

Differential Dx

- Cystitis
- Interstitial cystitis
- Foreign body
- Benign polyp

Presentation/Signs & Symptoms

- Gross or microscopic hematuria is the most common presentation
- Dysuria
- Frequency
- May be asymptomatic and discovered incidentally

Diagnostic Evaluation

- Urinalysis and urine culture to rule out infection
- Urine cytology
- Diagnostic cystoscopy will often visualize the tumor
- Upper tract evaluation (e.g., CT urography, IVP, retrograde pyelography) to rule out synchronous upper urinary tract carcinoma (will be present in 5% of patients with bladder carcinoma)
- Metastatic survey is indicated if the tumor invades the bladder wall
  - Bone scan to rule out bony metastases
  - CT scan of the abdomen and pelvis
  - Chest X-ray
  - Head CT if neurologic symptoms are present

Treatment/Management

- Transurethral resection is usually adequate initial management for superficial lesions
  - Biopsy should be done during resection; adequate tissue should be obtained to determine cell type, grade, depth of invasion, and associated satellite lesions such as carcinoma in situ (CIS)
- For superficial disease with high risk features (e.g., multiple lesions, high grade lesions, invasion of submucosa, associated CIS), adjuvant intravesical chemotherapy or immunotherapy is often used
- Invasive tumors (i.e., tumors that invade the muscularis layer of the bladder) require cystectomy with creation of a new bladder (generally using a piece of the ileum)

Prognosis/Complications

- Prognosis is excellent for superficial disease without high risk features; however, there is a high risk of recurrence, so close follow-up with repeat cystoscopic screening is necessary
- Superficial disease with high risk features will sometimes progress to invasive disease or will be refractory to conservative management; cystectomy may be required in these cases
- For invasive tumors that involve the muscularis layer, treatment with cystectomy carries a 60% 5-year survival rate
- Complications of bladder cancer include clot retention, ureteral obstruction, and metastatic spread to lymph nodes, bone, liver, and lung

100. Testicular Cancer

Etiology/Pathophysiology

- Most common solid tumor in men 20–34 years of age
  - Non-seminoma tumors are most common in 20–30s
  - Seminoma tumors are most common in 30–40s
- The greatest risk factor for testicular cancer is the presence of undescended testis at birth (cryptorchidism)
- Histologically, tumors are divided into non-seminoma (e.g., embryonal, teratoma, choriocarcinoma, yolk sack tumors) and seminoma; mixtures of multiple elements are common
- Most malignant testicular tumors arise from germ cells (90–95%); occasionally, tumors may arise from germ support cells, such as Leydig or Sertoli cells
- Metastasizes to nodes, then lungs, brain, bone, and/or liver

Differential Dx

- Epididymitis
- Testicular torsion
- Hydrocele
- Epididymal cyst
- Granulomatous orchitis
- Benign testicular mass

Presentation/Signs & Symptoms

- Painless lump or diffuse testicular enlargement is the most common presentation
- Acute onset of pain may signify a hemorrhage into the tumor
- Gynecomastia may infrequently occur due to release of paraneoplastic hormones by the tumor
- Hemoptysis may signal pulmonary metastases from a choriocarcinoma
- Abdominal pain or complaints may be secondary to retroperitoneal adenopathy
- Non-seminoma tumors tend to spread early; thus, these patients are more likely to present with metastatic disease

Diagnostic Evaluation

- In most cases, the diagnosis can be made on physical examination and confirmed by orchiectomy
  - Testicular biopsy or partial orchiectomy is not recommended
- Testicular ultrasound is the initial study of choice
- β-hCG and α-fetoprotein should be drawn before surgery to be used as markers of the primary disease
- After diagnosis, a metastatic workup should be done
  - CT scan of the chest, abdomen, and pelvis
  - CT of the head if neurologic symptoms are present

Treatment/Management

- Initial treatment consists of inguinal orchiectomy; subsequent treatment is determined by tumor histology and stage
- Early stage seminomas are usually treated with orchiectomy plus low dose external beam radiation to the ipsilateral nodal drainage
- Early stage non-seminomas are usually treated with orchiectomy plus either retroperitoneal lymphadenectomy or a surveillance protocol
- Advanced seminomas and non-seminomas are treated with platinum-based chemotherapy

Prognosis/Complications

- Outcomes for testicular cancer are among the best of all solid tumors—long-term cure rates exceed 90%, even with advanced disease
- Pure choriocarcinoma, though rare, is often rapidly fatal
- Possible long-term morbidities associated with treatment include infertility, retrograde ejaculation, lymphedema, or chylous ascites

101. Hydrocele

Etiology/Pathophysiology

- A painless scrotal mass caused by a collection of serous fluid between the parietal and visceral layers of the tunica vaginalis
- Most cases are idiopathic; however, underlying testicular pathology (e.g., testicular tumor, epididymitis) must be ruled out
- In children, a communicating hydrocele secondary to a patent processus vaginalis (a persistent embryonic peritoneal extension into the scrotum) may occur

Differential Dx

- Testicular neoplasm
- Epididymal cyst (spermatocele)
- Edema of Dartos (scrotal wall)
- Inguinal hernia

Presentation/Signs & Symptoms

- A chronic, progressive, *painless* enlargement of the scrotum
- Occasionally, tenderness may be present secondary to minor trauma
- Communicating hydrocele may vary widely in size depending on body position and other factors

Diagnostic Evaluation

- History should evaluate for chronicity, pain, variability, and fever
- Physical exam can readily differentiate between scrotal edema, hernia, and hydrocele
- A bright flashlight will transilluminate the scrotum if a hydrocele is present
- Testicular ultrasound is indicated if underlying testicular pathology is suspected

Treatment/Management

- Asymptomatic cases do not require specific treatment
- Aspiration of the hydrocele with or without injection of a sclerosing agent may be curative
- Definitive management involves surgical drainage with excision of redundant tunica vaginalis

Prognosis/Complications

- Prognosis is excellent
- Reaccumulation of the hydrocele fluid is common following aspiration procedures
- Infection is possible following needle aspiration
- Prolonged edema is common following surgical treatment

102. Acute Epididymitis

Etiology/Pathophysiology

- Infection or inflammation of the epididymis due to retrograde spread of bacteria through the urethra and bladder
- Most commonly caused by bacterial infection with *E. coli, Klebsiella, N. gonorrhea*, or Chlamydia
    - Chlamydia and gonorrhea are the most common causes in young males
    - *E. coli, Klebsiella*, and pseudomonas are more common in older patients
- Chemical epididymitis may be caused by reflux of urine from the urethra to the epididymis
- May rarely be drug induced (e.g., amiodarone)

Differential Dx

- Testicular torsion
- Orchitis
- Testicular tumor
- Torsion of appendix testis or appendix epididymis
- Testicular trauma

Presentation/Signs & Symptoms

- Gradual onset of unilateral scrotal pain
    - Usually occurs less acutely than testicular torsion
    - Increased pain when standing
    - Scrotal elevation decreases pain
- Exquisite tenderness of the epididymis
- Swelling of the epididymis, often with associated testicular swelling
- Fever may or may not be present
- Dysuria
- Nausea/vomiting is rare (as opposed to testicular torsion)
- May be found simultaneously with prostatitis and/or urinary tract infection

Diagnostic Evaluation

- History and physical examination are the keys to diagnosis
    - Differentiate epididymitis from testicular torsion (e.g., chronicity of symptoms, age of patient, presence of nausea, elevation of testis)
    - Edema and tenderness of the epididymis is diagnostic of epididymitis
- Urinalysis may or may not reveal pyuria
- Urine culture is indicated if pyuria is present on urinalysis
- Testicular ultrasound may be done in equivocal cases

Treatment/Management

- In the absence of specific culture results, administer antibiotics to cover the most common organisms for the age of presentation
    - In young, sexually active males, treat with doxycycline or a flouoroquinolone
    - *E. coli* predominates in older males; thus, trimethoprim-sulfamethoxazole is an additional choice
- Febrile patients or those with concomitant urosepsis may require hospital admission for IV antibiotics
- In patients with severe edema or those who do not respond to IV therapy, a high index of suspicion for testicular abscess is necessary (evaluate with a testicular ultrasound)
- Orchiectomy may occasionally be necessary in cases refractory to antibiotic therapy

Prognosis/Complications

- Most cases recover completely without sequellae
- Occasional cases will progress to testicular abscess
- Chronic epididymitis/chronic orchialgia may result in impairment of fertility

103. Testicular Torsion

Etiology/Pathophysiology

- Rotation of the testicle around the spermatic cord, thereby acutely compromising blood flow to the involved testis
- Untreated torsion results in testicular infarction in a matter of hours
- Most common in early adolescence
- Many cases present following trauma
- Associated with the "bell clapper" deformity, wherein the testicle rotates freely within the tunica vaginalis rather than being tethered

Differential Dx

- Epididymitis
- Viral or other orchitis
- Torsion of appendix testis
- Testicular neoplasm
- Strangulated inguinal hernia

Presentation/Signs & Symptoms

- The most common presentation is an adolescent who wakes up in the morning with testicular pain and vomiting
- Acute onset of testicular pain (as opposed to epididymitis, which has a more gradual onset)
- Nausea/vomiting is common
- Physical exam is generally characteristic for torsion
    - Diffuse testicular tenderness
    - High riding testicle
    - Prehn's sign: Elevation of the testis causes increased pain
    - Palpable knot in cord
    - Absent cremasteric reflex

Diagnostic Evaluation

- Due to the acute onset and rapid progression to testicular infarction, a suspicious history and physical exam is sufficient in many cases to recommend surgical exploration
- Urinalysis is usually normal in testicular torsion; pyuria generally indicates epididymitis
- Testicular ultrasound with Doppler blood flow study or radionuclide testicular scanning may be used in equivocal cases

Treatment/Management

- Torsion is a surgical emergency—treatment is best within 6 hours of symptom onset; by 24 hours, testicular infarction (necessitating orchiectomy) is very likely
- Manual detorsion by a urologist may be attempted prior to surgical exploration
- Surgical exploration of the scrotum with detorsion and orchidopexy of both testes
- Since the "bell clapper" deformity is bilateral, the patient is at risk for contralateral torsion; hence the recommendation for bilateral orchidopexy

Prognosis/Complications

- Prognosis is determined by the completeness of the torsion and length of time until detorsion
- In cases of complete torsion, best results are obtained if detorsion is performed within 6 hours of symptom onset
- Testis may undergo atrophy after detorsion

104. Acute Urinary Retention

Etiology/Pathophysiology

- Inability to void is usually due to an outlet obstruction
- The acute episode is precipitated by some factor that increases outlet resistance (e.g., clot, α-adrenergics, trauma, anal surgery) or diminishes detrusor function (e.g., anesthesia, anticholinergics, antihistamines)
- Causes of physical obstruction include benign prostatic hyperplasia (most common), urolithiasis, pelvic surgery, pelvic malignancy, prostate cancer, pregnancy, trauma, blood clots, phimosis or meatal stenosis, and infection
- Neurogenic causes include anesthesics (most common), diabetes, herniated disc, spinal cord injury or compression, medications (e.g., α-agonists, β-agonists, antihistamines, dicyclomine, diazepam, tricyclics, anticholinergics), multiple sclerosis, myasthenia gravis, Parkinson's disease, brain tumor, and cerebrovascular accident
- Results in increasing tubular pressures, leading to a progressive decrease in glomerular filtration rate (GFR) and, eventually, compromised renal perfusion

Differential Dx

- Intravascular volume depletion
- Acute renal failure
- Aortic aneurysm
- Pregnancy
- Pelvic or renal malignancy
- Uterine leiomyoma
- Ruptured bladder or urethra

Presentation/Signs & Symptoms

- Inability to void
- Change in urinary patterns (e.g., nocturia, polyuria, hesitancy, urgency, or difficulty starting stream)
- Significant abdominal, suprapubic, flank, or back pain is typically present secondary to distension
- Slowly progressive processes (e.g., tumors, BPH) may present without pain
- Distended, tender bladder on abdominal exam
- Rectal or pelvic exam may demonstrate enlarged pelvic structures, especially the prostate

Diagnostic Evaluation

- History should focus on BPH, prior procedures, strictures, sexual history, medications (e.g., cold remedies, antidepressants), and recent voiding pattern
- Physical exam should include percussion of bladder and prostate exam (extremely tender prostate may reflect acute prostatitis necessitating suprapubic tube placement)
- Look for signs of renal insufficiency and fluid overload (e.g., delirium, dyspnea, rales, edema, weight gain)
- Electrolyte disorders are often present (e.g., hyponatremia, hyperkalemia, acidosis)
- Urinalysis may reveal hematuria, pyuria, or crystalluria and will also rule out infection
- Post-void residual >125 cc is abnormal
- Imaging studies (helical CT scan, renal ultrasound, and/or intravenous pyelography) may be used to rule out causes of obstruction

Treatment/Management

- Place a Foley catheter to drain the bladder
  - If BPH is present, use a larger catheter
  - If negotiating the prostate is difficult, use a coudé catheter with the angled tip pointing up
  - If a stricture is present, use a smaller catheter
  - If unable to catheterize, consult urology for dilation, cystoscopic placement, or suprapubic tube placement
- Monitor bladder drainage
  - Allow urine to drain a liter at a time to avoid rapid emptying of the bladder, which can result in decompression hemorrhagic cystitis or a vasovagal response
  - Observe for post-obstructive diuresis
- Correct electrolyte and volume disturbances
- Definitive therapy may require prostate surgery, percutaneous nephrostomy tube, or cystoscopy with ureteral stent placement

Prognosis/Complications

- Complications include acute renal failure, transient gross hematuria, and post-obstructive diuresis
- Post-obstructive diuresis involves the loss of significant fluid after the relief of a chronic obstruction (due to transient tubule dysfunction); often results in volume, blood pressure, and electrolyte imbalances

105. Urinary Incontinence

Etiology/Pathophysiology

- Stress incontinence: Loss of urine associated with a rise in intra-abdominal pressure (e.g., coughing, lifting, bending, exercising)
  - More common in females with a history of vaginal childbirth due to a weakened pelvic floor
  - In men, it is most common following prostatectomy
- Urge incontinence (overactive bladder): Loss of urine due to hyperactivity of the detrusor muscle
  - Most cases are age-related and idiopathic
  - May occur secondary to loss of cortical inhibition of the micturition reflex (e.g., stroke, Parkinson's disease)
  - Local bladder etiologies include bladder tumors, stones, and infections
- Overflow incontinence: Loss of urine due to excess urine storage, either due to an atonic bladder (e.g., diabetic neuropathy, pelvic surgery, anticholinergic medications) or a bladder outlet obstruction (e.g., BPH, prostate cancer, strictures)
- Total incontinence: Constant loss of urine due to sphincter damage (e.g., post-prostatectomy) or an embryonic abnormality

Differential Dx

- Vesicovaginal fistula
- Colorectal fistula

Presentation/Signs & Symptoms

- Stress incontinence: History of incontinence following maneuvers that increase intra-abdominal pressure (e.g., coughing, lifting, bending, exercising)
- Urge incontinence: Patient is unable to sustain continence due to frequent urges to void ("cannot get to toilet in time")
- Overflow incontinence: Patient notices voiding small volumes of urine and notices bladder is full even after voiding (e.g., feeling of fullness, increased abdominal girth, suprapubic discomfort)
- Total incontinence: Absolutely no control of urine; urine just runs constantly
- Excoriation/skin care issues
- Patient may smell of urine

Diagnostic Evaluation

- History should focus on associated voiding symptoms, bowel function, fluid intake, medications, prior pelvic and abdominal surgery, and number of pads/day
- Patients should be instructed to complete a voiding diary prior to office visit
- Physical examination should include a pelvic exam in women (looking for cystocele and motion at the bladder neck), leakage with Valsalva, and neurologic evaluation; filling the bladder prior to exam is helpful
- Labs should include a urinalysis, blood glucose, BUN/creatinine, and urine culture
- Post-void residual can be evaluated by catheterization or ultrasound; will be elevated in overflow incontinence
- Cystoscopy is indicated for hematuria or persistent pyuria to rule out tumor or fistula
- Fluorourodynamic testing is indicated in difficult cases

Treatment/Management

- Stress incontinence is treated surgically to elevate and suspend the bladder and bladder neck
  - Surgical options include pubovaginal sling or transvaginal suspension
  - Intra-urethral collagen injection may be helpful
  - Medical treatment (α-adrenergics or estrogen preparations) may be helpful in mild cases
- Urge incontinence is generally treated medically
  - Anticholinergics (e.g., oxybutynin, tolterodine) are often effective to improve detrusor instability
  - Other treatments include behavioral modification, biofeedback, and sacral nerve stimulators
- Overflow incontinence
  - Atonic bladder is treated with intermittent self-catheterization or nerve stimulator
  - In cases of obstruction, surgical correction may allow preservation of adequate voiding

Prognosis/Complications

- Involuntary loss of urine afflicts millions, costs billions to manage, and is associated with significant psychologic morbidity and social impairment
- Urge incontinence: Medical management is successful in >80% of cases
- Stress incontinence: Sling procedures are successful in >80% of cases
- Overflow incontinence: If not managed properly, may lead to renal failure

106. Urolithiasis

Etiology/Pathophysiology

- Most often due to increased concentrations of stone-forming material in the urine, either from increased excretion or decreased urinary volume
- Common in patients with urinary stasis (e.g., bladder outlet obstruction) and/or chronic infection
- Calcium stones are the etiology in >75% of cases (calcium oxalate is the most common type, followed by calcium phosphate)
  - Due to hypercalciuria (secondary to excessive intestinal absorption of calcium), hyperparathyroidism, excess vitamin D, or bone metastases
  - Hyperoxaluria results from over consumption of oxalate rich foods, short gut syndromes, and inborn metabolic disorders
  - Ironically, high dietery calcium intake may decrease the risk of stone formation as it forms ligands with oxalate and phosphate
- Uric acid stones are associated with low urine pH (e.g., chronic diarrhea) and hyperuricosuria (e.g., gout, myeloproliferative states)
  - May occur with severe dehydration despite normal uric acid levels
- Struvite stones (composed of magnesium ammonium phosphate) occur in patients with chronic UTIs caused by urea splitting bacteria (e.g., Proteus)
  - Often fills the entire renal collecting system, resulting in "staghorn" calculi

Differential Dx

- Pyelonephritis
- Ectopic pregnancy
- Pelvic inflammatory disease
- Renal cell carcinoma
- Flank or abdominal wall trauma
- Pancreatitis
- Biliary colic
- Appendicitis
- Abdominal aortic aneurysm

Presentation/Signs & Symptoms

- Severe, acute, colicky flank pain
- Pain may radiate to the lower abdomen, groin, testicles, or perineum
- Nausea/vomiting
- Diaphoresis
- Hematuria
- Costovertebral angle tenderness

Diagnostic Evaluation

- Clinical presentation is highly predictive, especially in patients with a past history of urolithiasis
- Urinalysis will reveal hematuria, unless a complete urinary tract obstruction is present
- Non-contrast abdominal CT is the test of choice to detect stones and urinary tract obstructions
  - Uric acid stones are the only radiolucent stones; thus they will not show up on X-ray but are opaque on CT
- Strain the urine for stones and send to lab for analysis of stone composition

Treatment/Management

- Small stones (<5 mm) will often pass spontaneously
- Immediate treatment is indicated if the patient presents with fever, renal failure, intractable pain, persistent nausea, or UTI
- Stones in the kidney are often treated with extracorporeal shock wave lithotripsy (ESWL)
  - Large stones and struvite stones are best treated by percutaneous removal or (rarely) open pyelolithotomy
  - Uric acid stones can be dissolved by hydration and urinary alkalinization with potassium citrate
- Stones in the ureters are treated with ESWL, ureteroscopy, or intracorporeal laser lithotripsy
- Stones in the bladder are often treated by stolithalopaxy with endoscopic stone crushing and extraction of fragments
  - Very large or hard stones may require a small open cystostomy for removal

Prognosis/Complications

- Recurrence is common; patients who tend to form stones should be instructed in methods of stone prevention
  - General measures include increased fluid intake, restriction of animal protein and salt, avoidance of oxalate-containing foods (e.g., tea, dark greens, chocolate), and consumption of citrate (e.g., lemons)
  - Potassium citrate is a good supplement for most calcium stone formers and those with uric acid and cysteine stones
  - A complete metabolic analysis and specific medication regimen may be necessary in severe cases

107. Hematuria

Etiology/Pathophysiology

- Distinguish gross (visible) hematuria from microscopic hematuria
- Ruling out the presence of a neoplasm is the primary goal of the subsequent evaluation (underlying malignancy is present in 10% of cases)
- Urinary tract infection is the most common cause
- May originate anywhere along the urinary tract
  - Kidney etiologies include trauma, glomerulonephritis, nephrolithiasis, tumors, infarction, and polycystic kidney disease
  - Ureteral etiologies include urolithiasis and tumors
  - Bladder etiologies include trauma, urolithiasis, cystitis, and tumors
  - Prostate etiologies include prostate cancer, prostatitis, and varices (in BPH)
  - Urethral etiologies include trauma (including Foley catheter placement), urolithiasis, and tumors
- May occur in patients with generalized bleeding disorders (e.g., excessive anticoagulation, hematologic conditions)

Differential Dx

- Myoglobinuria
- Bilirubinuria (liver failure)

Presentation/Signs & Symptoms

- Painless hematuria suggests tumor or BPH
- Irritative symptoms (e.g., dysuria, nocturia) suggests inflammation (e.g., UTI) or bladder cancer
- Colicky pain suggests urolithiasis
- Lower abdominal pain suggests urinary retention
- Fever suggests pyelonephritis or severe cystitis
- Hematuria throughout the urinary stream suggests pathology above the bladder neck
- Hematuria at the end of the urinary stream suggests a prostatic source
- Hematuria at the start of urination suggests a urethral source

Diagnostic Evaluation

- Urinalysis is the initial study
  - Dysmorphic RBCs, proteinuria, and/or casts suggest renal disease
  - Pyuria indicates an inflammatory etiology (e.g., UTI)
  - Crystals suggests urolithiasis
- Urine culture and sensitivity (before beginning therapy)
- Cytology should be evaluated in smokers and if transitional cells are noted on urinalysis
- Upper tract imaging may be indicated based on presentation
  - Ultrasound, CT, or IVP will evaluate for painless microscopic hematuria
  - Non-contrast CT is indicated if a stone is suspected
  - Retrograde pyelogram may be indicated for obstruction
- Cystoscopy must be done if bladder cancer is suspected (e.g., in smokers or if other etiologies have been ruled out) and in cases of recurrent UTIs

Treatment/Management

- Treatment depends on the underlying cause
- See related entries in this section for individual treatments of specific disorders

Prognosis/Complications

- Close follow-up is necessary in older patients due to high risk of underlying malignancies

Thoracic Surgery

Section 12

JASON J. LAMB, MD

108. Thoracic Anatomy, Facts, and Pearls

- The lungs are responsible for gas exchange at the alveolar-capillary membrane, thereby eliminating carbon dioxide waste and delivering oxygen to deoxygenated hemoglobin
- The majority of lung diseases produce deleterious effects by altering delivery of air, altering delivery of blood, inhibiting efficient gas exchange, or some combination of these effects

Thoracic Anatomy

- The respiratory system consists of the nose, nasal passages, nasopharynx, larynx, trachea, bronchi, and lungs
- Associated thoracic structures with integral roles are the bony and muscular thorax, the pleura, and the mediastinum
- The mediastinum includes the trachea, esophagus, thymus, heart, great vessels, mediastinal fat, and mediastinal lymph nodes
- Pleura include the visceral pleura on the lung surface and parietal pleura on the inner thoracic wall, with an intervening potential space

Pulmonary Anatomy

- The lungs include the segmental bronchi, bronchioles, and alveoli
- The right lung is larger and has three lobes (upper, middle, and lower)
- The left lung has two lobes (upper and lower)
- The oblique (major) fissure divides the upper and lower lobes on both sides
- The horizontal (minor) fissure is present only on the right side and separates the upper and middle lobes
- Each lobe is then divided into segments (10 on the right and 8 on the left)
- The lingula is a segment within the left upper lobe
- The trachea has anterior cartilaginous rings and a posterior membranous portion
- Mainstem bronchi arise at the seventh thoracic vertebra
- The right mainstem bronchus is shorter and less angled than the right—foreign body aspiration is more common into the right mainstem bronchus due to its steeper angle
- Bronchioles are ciliated, lack cartilage, contain smooth muscle, and deliver air to the alveoli
- Pulmonary gas exchange occurs at the alveolus

Blood Supply and Lymphatics

- The pulmonary artery carries deoxygenated blood to the lungs
- The pulmonary vein carries oxygenated blood to the left atrium
- The pulmonary artery arises to the left of the aorta
- Typically, a superior and inferior pulmonary vein on each side return pulmonary blood to the left atrium
- Bronchial arterial flow supplies most of the lung tissue with oxygenated blood
- Bronchial arteries arise from the systemic circulation (usually aorta and intercostals) and comprise 1% of cardiac output
- Lymphatic drainage is typically to intraparenchymal, bronchopulmonary, interlobar, hilar, and then mediastinal nodes

109. Pleural Effusion

Etiology/Pathophysiology

- Excess fluid in the pleural space
- Due to either excess pleural fluid formation or diminished fluid removal by the pleural lymphatics
    - Pleural fluid is formed at approximately 0.01 mL/kg/hr in the capillaries of the visceral and parietal pleura, the interstitial space of the lung, and the peritoneal cavity
    - Pleural fluid is cleared by lymphatics at rate of 0.3 mL/kg/hr
- Transudative effusions are caused by systemic factors that influence the production of pleural fluid; however, the pleural fluid itself is normal
- Exudative effusions arise from pleural inflammation that causes increased capillary permeability or from obstruction of lymphatic drainage
- 1 million cases/year in the U.S.

Differential Dx

- Transudative causes include CHF, cirrhosis, nephrotic syndrome, peritoneal dialysis, SVC obstruction, myxedema, pulmonary embolus, and sarcoidosis
- Exudative causes include neoplasms, infections, post-operative, esophageal perforation, diaphragmatic hernia, pancreatic disease, collagen vascular disease, asbestosis, chylothorax, hemothorax, thoracic radiation exposure, trapped lung, and drug-induced pleural disease (e.g., amiodarone)

Presentation/Signs & Symptoms

- Shortness of breath
- Dyspnea on exertion
- Cough
- Pleuritic chest pain
- Tachypnea
- Orthopnea
- Physical exam demonstrates absent or diminished breath sounds, dullness to percussion, and rales on affected side
- Hypoxia and/or hypercapnea

Diagnostic Evaluation

- Detailed history to identify transudative or exudative causes
- Upright PA and lateral chest X-ray will a reveal blunted costophrenic angle (up to 500 mL may not be seen on upright CXR)
- Lateral decubitus chest X-ray, chest CT scan, or ultrasound will all demonstrate free pleural fluid
- Further workup indicated for large effusions (>10 mm space between lung and chest wall on decubitus chest X-ray)
- Diagnostic thoracentesis is performed for pleural fluid analysis to determine transudate versus exudate
    - Evaluate pleural fluid for pH, glucose, amylase, LDH, cytology, differential cell counts, and microbiologic cultures
    - Elevated pleural fluid to serum ratios of protein or LDH suggest exudative effusion

Treatment/Management

- Thoracentesis may be therapeutic
- Ultrasound-guided thoracentesis should be used for localized effusion
- Closed tube thoracostomy is used for empyema, hemothorax, and recurrent pleural effusions
    - Tube thoracostomy is connected to a closed water seal system rather than suction to prevent pneumothorax
    - Tube is usually removed only when drainage <100 cc/day
- Pleurodesis with doxycycline or talc is used to obliterate the pleural space in cases of intractable pleural effusion

Prognosis/Complications

- Prognosis depends on the underlying disease
- Pneumothorax may occur with thoracentesis
- Empyema may occur with contamination of the pleural space
- Hemothorax may occur if an intercostal vessel is injured
- Re-expansion pulmonary edema may occur with thoracentesis >1500 cc
- Rare cases of ARDS may occur following large volume drainage of chronic effusion

110. Empyema

Etiology/Pathophysiology

- A collection of pus in the pleural cavity that occurs when bacteria invade the normally sterile pleural space
- Caused by a contaminated pleural effusion or post-surgical infection
- Stages of development
  - Stage 1: Exudative effusion, uncomplicated parapneumonic effusion
  - Stage 2: Bacterial invasion resulting in a fibrinopurulent proliferation
  - Stage 3: Organization of collagen, lung entrapment, "peel" formation
- In the modern antibiotic era, *Peptostreptococcus, Staphylococcus epidermidis, Streptococcus viridans*, and anaerobes are the most common causative organisms of parapneumonic empyema
- Patients with pneumonia due to anaerobic and gram-negative bacteria are much more likely to develop empyema; however, patients with streptococcal pneumonia are unlikely to develop empyema

Differential Dx

- Uncomplicated pneumonia with a sterile parapneumonic effusion
- Uncomplicated pleural effusion
- COPD exacerbation
- Congestive heart failure
- Bronchitis
- Atelectasis
- Trapped lung
- Lung abscess
- Prior pulmonary resection
- Diaphragmatic hernia
- Paraesophageal hernia
- Pulmonary embolism
- Acute pancreatitis
- Tuberculosis

Presentation/Signs & Symptoms

- Shortness of breath
- Fever
- Cough
- Chest discomfort
- History of previous pneumonia, recent thoracic trauma, or recent surgery
- May have subtle progression or recurrence of septic pneumonia course
- Physical exam often demonstrates tachypnea, tachycardia, hypoxia, and anxiety
- Dullness to percussion and diminished chest wall motion on the affected side
- Clubbing and shrunken chest wall occur with chronic disease

Diagnostic Evaluation

- Chest X-ray (PA and lateral followed by bilateral decubitus views) may show the classic "inverted D" in the posterior sulcus on lateral view
- Chest CT will distinguish empyema from lung abscess and other parenchymal disease
- Ultrasound is similar in efficacy to CT at visualizing pleural fluid; however, it is not as accurate at identifying parenchymal abnormalities
- CT-guided thoracentesis is very accurate and is often diagnostic (ultrasound-guided thoracentesis is also used)
  - Will differentiate an effusion from empyema
  - Turbid or purulent fluid is diagnostic of empyema
  - Low pH, low glucose, and high LDH suggests bacterial infection
  - Differential cell counts, gram stain, and culture
- Blood, sputum, and empyema fluid cultures

Treatment/Management

- Administer appropriate antibiotic therapy to control infection and sepsis
- Thin, less purulent fluid may be completely removed during diagnostic thoracentesis
- Closed tube thoracostomy is the first step in treating acute empyema; the tube may be removed once drainage is <50 cc/day
- Video-assisted thoracoscopy (VATS) is now the primary modality for complicated empyema
- Open thoracotomy or minithoracotomy with tube drainage is indicated for large space empyema requiring prolonged drainage

Prognosis/Complications

- Good prognosis if identified and drained early
- Mortality approaches 15% for late diagnosed cases
- Complications may include sepsis, trapped lung, bronchopleural fistula from visceral pleural necrosis, osteomyelitis of the ribs or spine from parietal pleural necrosis, mediastinitis, esophageal fistula, pericarditis, or brain abscess

111. Pneumothorax

Etiology/Pathophysiology

- Air in the pleural space, resulting in lung collapse
- Spontaneous pneumothorax is not usually associated with precipitating activity; most commonly occurs due to rupture of a subpleural bleb
- Acquired pneumothorax is due to trauma (e.g., chest wall trauma with rib fracture, barotrauma, central venous catheter insertion)
- Tension pneumothorax occurs when air enters the pleural space during each breath but the air is unable to be released during expiration; results in significant increase in intrapleural pressure and impedes venous return to the heart, resulting in cardiovascular collapse
- Open pneumothorax occurs with penetrating chest trauma and open communication of the pleural space to the outside

Differential Dx

- Asthma or COPD exacerbation
- Congestive heart failure
- Myocardial infarction
- Pulmonary embolism
- Aspiration
- Tracheal or bronchial foreign body
- Non-ruptured giant bullae
- Pneumonia
- Pleurisy
- Ruptured diaphragm
- Free air due to perforated abdominal viscus

Presentation/Signs & Symptoms

- Sudden onset of shortness of breath, cough, and pleuritic chest pain
- Diminished or absent breath sounds, hyperresonance to percussion, and diminished tactile fremitus on the affected side
- Tachycardia, diaphoresis, hypotension, and pallor occur with tension pneumothorax
- Tracheal shift to uninvolved side in tension pneumothorax

Diagnostic Evaluation

- History and physical examination
  - Due to the rapid decompensation that occurs with tension pneumothorax, clinical suspicion is sufficient to proceed with immediate needle decompression
- Upright chest X-ray is usually diagnostic
  - Thin radiolucent pleural line
  - Absence of vascular lung markings peripheral to the radiolucent line
  - Tracheal deviation to the opposite side
  - Lateral decubitus film with the suspected side up may be helpful for indeterminate cases
  - Exhalation chest X-ray may reveal mild cases
- Chest CT is very sensitive but only used if X-ray is inconclusive

Treatment/Management

- Observation alone for small pneumothorax
- Needle aspiration or percutaneous catheter drainage in mild/moderate cases
- Tube thoracostomy for large pneumothoraces >30%
  - Connect to a closed water seal system initially
  - If lung does not re-expand, connect tube to suction at −20 cm of pressure
  - Heimlich valve may be used for outpatient management
- Indications for surgical treatment include recurrent spontaneous pneumothorax, persistent air leak >5–7 days, or if subject to barometric changes
- Surgical correction (thoracoscopy or thoracotomy) involves excision of the offending bleb and promotion of pleural adhesion via physical or chemical pleurodesis and/or parietal pleurectomy

Prognosis/Complications

- Operative intervention is effective in >95% cases
- Operative complications include pleuritic pain, persistent air leak, post-thoracotomy pain syndrome, wound infection, and post-op empyema
- 20–50% risk of recurrence for non-surgically treated spontaneous pneumothorax

112. Lung Abscess

Etiology/Pathophysiology

- Usually a single, cavitary lesion of localized pus contained within the lung parenchyma due to necrosis of lung tissue
- Most cases result from aspiration of oral secretions
    - Risk factors for aspiration include alcohol abuse, seizure disorders, esophageal disorders, neuromuscular disorders, periodontal disease, intubation, and tube feedings
    - Most frequently caused by oral anaerobes (e.g., Bacteroides), *Staphylococcus aureus,* or *Streptococcus pneumoniae*
    - Develops 7–14 days after aspiration
    - Generally occurs in the superior segments of the right and left lower lobes or the lateral posterior segment of the right upper lobe
- Other causes of lung abscess include pulmonary embolism with infarction, chest trauma, or obstruction
- Defined as acute if <6 weeks duration

Differential Dx

- Other cavitary lung lesions
    - Tuberculosis
    - Fungal infection
    - Cancer
    - Vasculitis
    - Wegener's granulomatosis
    - Acute necrotizing pneumonia
    - Lymphoma
    - Bronchiectasis

Presentation/Signs & Symptoms

- Intermittent fevers
- Purulent sputum
- Foul-smelling breath
- Coarse breath sounds
- Toxic appearance

Diagnostic Evaluation

- Detailed history of dental work, antecedent pneumonia, and aspiration risk
- CBC will reveal leukocytosis but blood cultures are rarely positive
- Obtain sputum cultures to identify causative organisms
- Chest X-ray will reveal a complex air-fluid level, often seen in dependent lung zones (e.g., superior lower lobe or posterior upper lobes)
- CT scan is helpful to define and localize the abscess
- Flexible bronchoscopy will rule out an endobronchial mass and allow for cytologic washings

Treatment/Management

- Administer broad-spectrum antibiotics until definitive cultures are available
- Once causative organism is identified, begin a 6–8 week course of appropriate antibiotic coverage
- Postural drainage by chest physiotherapy or bronchoscopy may be sufficient
- CT-guided percutaneous catheter drainage is reserved for abscesses that do not resolve with postural drainage and antibiotic therapy
- Tube thoracostomy or open pneumonostomy are reserved for septic patients or when percutaneous measures fail
- Surgical resection is required urgently for bleeding, empyema, or bronchopleural fistula
- Consider surgical resection for persistent abscess (>8 weeks), chronic complications, or suspicion of carcinoma

Prognosis/Complications

- Medical therapy is the rule; surgical intervention is reserved for complicated cases
- With the advent of percutaneous drainage, only 10% of cases require surgery
- Acute complications include bronchopleural fistula, empyema, and bleeding, requiring immediate surgical resection
- Chronic complications include persistent infection, persistent abscess >6 cm after 8 weeks of therapy, recurrent empyema, and bronchopleural fistula

113. Benign Lung Tumors

Etiology/Pathophysiology

- May be epithelial, mesodermal, or endothelial in origin
- May arise in the central bronchi or in the peripheral lung
- >50% of solitary pulmonary nodules found on CT scan are benign
- Prevalence is increasing due to improvements in imaging sensitivity
- Lesions in young non-smokers are more likely to be benign
- Benign non-neoplastic lesions are more common than benign neoplasms
  - Benign non-neoplastic lesions include AV malformations, infectious granuloma, abscess, bronchogenic cyst, pulmonary infarction, rounded atelectasis, sequestration
  - Benign neoplasms include hamartoma (common), fibroma, chondroma, lipoma, granular myoblastoma

Differential Dx

- Lung malignancy
- Pulmonary metastases
- Mediastinal tumors
- Pleural base tumors
- Atelectasis

Presentation/Signs & Symptoms

- Lesions are usually asymptomatic and found incidentally on imaging
- Stridor, wheezing, and dyspnea are common only if the lesion is endobronchial and central
- Dyspnea occurs with AV malformations secondary to shunting
- Hemoptysis is also common with AV malformations

Diagnostic Evaluation

- History and physical exam are not usually helpful, as most lesions are asymptomatic
- Most nodules are diagnosed on chest radiographs
- High resolution CT scan is now the cornerstone for evaluation and diagnosis of benign pulmonary nodules
  - Benign lesions are more likely to be calcified, stable over time, smooth-bordered, smaller, and very high density (due to calcium content) or very low density (due to fat content)
- Positron emission tomography (PET) is becoming more useful as a diagnostic tool (high sensitivity but moderate specificity)
- Tissue evaluation for definitive diagnosis can be accomplished by sputum cytology, bronchoscopy with biopsy, CT-guided percutaneous biopsy, video-assisted thoracoscopic (VATS) biopsy, or thoracotomy with open biopsy

Treatment/Management

- Patients thought to be at low risk for neoplasm may be periodically surveyed via CT scanning
  - If change in lesion appearance is noted on CT scan, biopsy or resection is indicated
  - Continue periodic repeat CT scans if no change
- High risk lesions require biopsy or resection
  - Non-surgical biopsy may be accomplished by CT-guided fine needle aspiration (for low or moderate risk lesions) or bronchoscopic biopsy (for endobronchial lesions)
  - Video-assisted thoracoscopic surgery (VATS) with wedge resection; if tissue proves to be malignant, lobectomy may then be indicated
  - Initial thoracotomy is indicated for highly suspicious lesions
- Once a lesion is confirmed to be benign by tissue diagnosis, no further follow-up is necessary

Prognosis/Complications

- Prognosis is obviously excellent with truly benign lesions; however, failure to diagnose a malignant lesion may result in significant mortality
- FNA is generally tolerated well but may be complicated by pneumothorax or hemothorax formation
- Thoracotomy may be complicated by post-thoracotomy pain (common), persistent air leak (<10%), post-surgical empyema (<2%), or wound infection (<5%)

114. Primary Lung Cancer

Etiology/Pathophysiology

- Second most common malignancy (170,000 new cases/year in U.S.)
- Most common cause of cancer-related death (25% of all cancer deaths)
- Smoking is the primary etiology in >80% of lung cancers
- 15% of smokers will develop lung cancer
- Small cell lung cancers (SCLC) tend to grow rapidly and metastasize early
  - Small cell carcinoma (20% of lung cancers): Undifferentiated, centrally located, and usually presents with advanced disease
  - Carcinoid tumors (5% of lung cancers): Differentiated, neuroendocrine tumors that arise from bronchi, centrally located, and rarely metastasize
  - Neuroendocrine carcinoma or atypical carcinoid (1% of lung cancers): Less differentiated, more peripheral, and more aggressive
- Non-small cell lung cancers (NSCLC)
  - Adenocarcinoma (40% of lung cancers): Glandular, peripheral, nodal/distant metastases are common, non-smokers/women
  - Bronchoalveolar cell carcinoma (2% of lung cancers): Glandular adenocarcinoma, variable, non-smokers/women
  - Squamous cell carcinoma (25% of lung cancers): Usually central, usually localized with regional nodal spread, may be cavitary
  - Large cell carcinoma (7% of lung cancer): More peripheral

Differential Dx

- Benign lung lesions
  - Non-neoplastic lesions (e.g., granuloma, atelectasis, abscess, AV malformation)
  - Benign neoplastic lesions (e.g., hamartoma)
- Pulmonary metastasis
- Other malignancy

Presentation/Signs & Symptoms

- 90–95% of patients are symptomatic (versus <50% of patients with benign lesions)
- Cough, dyspnea, wheezing, and hemoptysis are common presentations
- Fever (postobstructive pneumonia)
- Pleural effusion and chest wall pain may indicate regional spread
- Paraneoplastic syndromes occur in 10–15% of cases, usually SCLC (e.g., SIADH, Eaton-Lambert syndrome, Trousseau's syndrome, ectopic PTH)
- Less common presentations include superior vena cava syndrome, Horner's syndrome (miosis, ptosis, anhidrosis), Pancoast's tumor, phrenic nerve/vagus nerve/esophagus involvement

Diagnostic Evaluation

- History and physical exam
- Chest X-ray has a limited detection of lesions <7 mm
- CT scan is the cornerstone of evaluation to determine tumor size and extent, mediastinal node involvement, and liver/adrenal metastases
- CT or MRI of brain and bone scan to evaluate metastases
- Pre-operative histologic diagnosis by sputum cytology, bronchoscopic biopsy (central), fluoroscopic FNA, or CT-guided biopsy (peripheral)
- Staging of mediastinum with mediastinoscopy, CT-guided biopsy, PET scan, or bronchoscopic directed biopsy
- Pre-operative determination of whether the patient will be able to tolerate lobectomy or pneumonectomy
  - Pulmonary function studies and differential V/Q scans (calculated postoperative FEV_1 should be >0.8)
  - ABG showing pCO_2 >45 or pO_2 <60 suggest a high risk for complications

Treatment/Management

- SCLC management is almost exclusively non-surgical
  - Responds well to combination chemotherapy
  - Radiation to symptomatic sites for palliation
  - Prophylactic brain radiation is often used as >80% of patients develop brain metastases
  - Surgery is indicated only for isolated lesions without metastases (rare)
- NSCLC
  - Stage I/II disease are resectable: Lobectomy is preferred but pneumonectomy, segmentectomy, and non-anatomic resections may be used; adjuvant chemotherapy increases survival
  - Surgery has limited or no role in stage III/IV disease; radiation treatment may be used palliatively
  - Primary and adjuvant chemotherapy (long-term response 5–15%)

Prognosis/Complications

- 15% overall 5-year survival for all lung cancers
  - NSCLC stage I: 60–70% 5-year survival
  - NSCLC stage II: 40% 5-year survival
  - NSCLC stage III/IV: <15% 5-year survival
  - Untreated SCLC survival <6 month
  - Chemotherapy-treated SCLC <10% 5-year survival (however, 50% of patients have an initial positive response)
- Complications of unresectable tumors include pleural effusion, post-obstructive pneumonia, airway obstruction, bronchopleural fistula, and metastases
- Complications of resected tumors include local or distant recurrence, empyema, bronchopleural fistula, and post-thoracotomy pain

115. Mediastinal Tumors

Etiology/Pathophysiology

- May be congenital, infectious, developmental, traumatic, or neoplastic
- Neurogenic tumors (23%) are the most common posterior compartment tumor
    - Include schwannoma, neurofibroma, ganglioneuroblastoma, neuroblastoma, pheochromocytoma, and paraganglioma
- Thymic tumors (19%) are the most common anterior compartment tumor
- Cysts (18%) are the most common visceral compartment tumor
- Lymphoma (12%) causes 50% of childhood mediastinal masses
- Germ cell tumors (12%) include teratomas, seminomas, and non-seminomatous germ cell tumors
- Miscellaneous cysts (8%) and mesenchymal tumors (8%) include thyroid goiter, thyroid cancer, parathyroid adenomas, bronchogenic cyst, pericardial cyst, aneurysm, and esophageal diverticula

Differential Dx

- Anterior mediastinum: Thymoma, germ cell tumors, lymphoma, lymphangioma, hemangioma, lipoma, fibroma, thymic cyst, aberrant thyroid, and parathyroid tumors
- Posterior mediastinum: Schwannoma, lymphoma, neurofibroma, ganglioneuroblastoma, neuroblastoma, pheochromocytoma
- Visceral mediastinum: Inclusion cyst, lymphoma, pericardial cyst, granuloma, hamartoma, mesothelial cyst, pheochromocytoma

Presentation/Signs & Symptoms

- Usually asymptomatic; however, symptoms are common in children
    - 95% of asymptomatic masses are benign
    - 50% of symptomatic masses are benign
- Cough, dyspnea, and stridor may occur due to compression
- Chest pain, pleural effusion, hoarseness, paraplegia, and back pain suggest invasive disease

Diagnostic Evaluation

- History and physical exam
- Chest X-ray is the cornerstone of diagnosis; 50% of mediastinal lesions are diagnosed by chest X-ray
- Spiral CT scan with contrast helps to determine features of the lesion
- Adjunctive tests may include MRI with angiography (for hemangioma), thyroid/parathyroid nuclear scanning, MIBG scanning (for pheochromocytoma), gallium scanning (for lymphoma), and serum markers (for germ cell tumors, thymoma)
- CT- or ultrasound-guided fine needle aspiration to evaluate histology of the lesion
- Tissue diagnosis may also be obtained via bronchoscopy, esophagoscopy, mediastinoscopy, mediastinotomy (Chamberlain procedure), thoracostomy, or (rarely) thoracotomy

Treatment/Management

- Benign neurogenic tumors are often observed in elderly or debilitated patients; resection is indicated in young patients or those with potentially malignant lesions
- Thymomas are treated by resection with postoperative radiation
- Lymphoma is treated by radiation and/or chemotherapy
- Germ cell tumors
    - Benign teratomas are resected
    - Malignant teratomas are usually widely metastatic at diagnosis
    - Seminomas are treated with radiation
    - Non-seminomatous tumors are treated with chemotherapy and resection of residual mass
- Miscellaneous cysts and mesenchymal tumors are usually resected

Prognosis/Complications

- Very good prognosis for resected benign lesions
- Chest X-ray is the mainstay of follow-up after resection
- Complications of fine needle aspiration include pneumothorax (20–25%), hemoptysis (5%), and nondiagnosis (20–40%)
- Mediastinoscopy can rarely result in tracheobronchial or vascular injury

116. Upper Respiratory Tumors

Etiology/Pathophysiology

- Bronchial and tracheal tumors are rare; however, bronchial tumors are 100 times more common than tracheal tumors
- Tracheal tumors more commonly occur in the mid-trachea in children and in the distal trachea in adults
- Chondroma is the most common benign tumor
- Respiratory hemangioma will commonly spontaneously regress
- Squamous cell carcinoma comprises 50% of all primary tracheal malignancies
  - Most common in the distal one-third of trachea
- Adenoid cystic carcinoma is slow growing but invasive to the submucosa
  - Most common in the proximal one-third of trachea
- Typical carcinoid behaves in a "benign" fashion
- Atypical carcinoid is more aggressive and has much greater malignant potential

Differential Dx

- Benign lesions include chondroma, papilloma, fibroma, hemangioma, granular cell tumor, lipoma, leiomyoma, hamartoma, and mucous gland adenoma
- Malignant lesions include squamous cell carcinoma (associated with hemoptysis), adenoid cystic carcinoma, carcinoid (typical versus atypical), small cell carcinoma, and adenocarcinoma

Presentation/Signs & Symptoms

- Shortness of breath occurs when two-thirds of the airway becomes obstructed
- Dyspnea on exertion
- Cough
- Wheezing
- Stridor
- Hemoptysis is indicative of carcinoma
- Dysphagia (uncommon)
- Physical exam may reveal cervical lymphadenopathy, inspiratory wheezing, and consolidative breath sounds suggestive of obstructive pneumonia

Diagnostic Evaluation

- Chest X-ray may reveal tracheal mass
- Bronchoscopy with biopsy is used for diagnosis, assessment of lesion characteristics, and evaluation of vocal cord function
- CT scan evaluates for length of lesion, mediastinal extent, compression, lumen size, tumor characteristics, and node involvement and aids in surgical planning
- MRI defines precise dimensions
- Barium esophogram should be administered if dysphagia is present
- Pulmonary function studies should be done to rule out an obstructive pattern

Treatment/Management

- Most benign lesions can be treated with bronchoscopic removal; recurrences are usually treated with laser ablation or photodynamic therapy
- Tracheal resection is reserved for malignant primary tumors or large benign tumors
  - Tracheal resection can be performed up to 4 cm in length safely
  - Mediastinal node involvement precludes resection
- Resection of malignant tumors should be followed by postoperative radiation
- Palliation for unresectable advanced disease should be attempted due to impending airway obstruction
  - Radiation therapy may be used in advanced malignant disease
  - Rigid and flexible bronchoscopy with photodynamic therapy, laser, bronchial stent, or brachytherapy techniques

Prognosis/Complications

- Most benign lesions carry an excellent prognosis following local endoscopic intervention
- Squamous cell carcinoma has a 40% 5-year survival following resection
- Adenoid cystic carcinoma has a 66% 5-year and 50% 10-year survival following resection
- Complications include recurrent pulmonary infection/pneumonia, hemoptysis, pneumothorax/pneumomediastinum, tracheal stenosis, airway obstruction, and bronchopleural fistula formation

117. Lung Transplantation

Etiology/Pathophysiology

- Common indications for lung transplantation
  - Obstructive lung disease (e.g., emphysema, which is the most common disease treated with lung transplantation)
  - Restrictive lung disease (e.g., idiopathic pulmonary fibrosis)
  - Cystic fibrosis
  - Pulmonary hypertension (e.g., primary pulmonary hypertension, Eisenmenger's syndrome)
- Unlike other solid organ transplants, no systemic arterial supply can be grafted because the bronchial artery anatomy is small, distant, and widely varied; thus, complications are common and are related to ischemia

Differential Dx

Presentation/Signs & Symptoms

Diagnostic Evaluation

- Indications for lung transplant: Age <60, life expectancy <18 months, exhausted medical/surgical options, ambulatory patient with rehabilitation potential, no contraindications to immunosuppresion, psychosocial support, and no contraindications
- Absolute contraindications: Acute illness, significant major organ disease, sepsis, uncontrolled neoplasm, current smoking, noncompliance, and psychiatric problems
- Relative contraindications: Age >65, nutritional depletion, osteoporosis, prior major cardiac or thoracic surgery, moderate non-pulmonary systemic disease, moderate CAD or LV dysfunction, or ongoing high dose corticosteroid use
- Only 25% of multiple organ donors qualify
- Donor indications: Age <55, ABO compatibility, clear chest X-ray, smoking <20 pack-years, no significant trauma or aspiration, size match, pO_2 >300 on 100% O_2, <5 cm H_2O PEEP

Treatment/Management

- Single (SLT) or double (DLT) lung transplantation
  - Single transplantation is more efficient use of organs in limited supply
  - Usually can be done without cardiopulmonary bypass
  - Intra-operative complications include technical anastomotic problems, phrenic injury, recurrent laryngeal injury, and myocardial infarction

Prognosis/Complications

- >70% 1-year survival; <50% 5-year survival
- Only a fraction of patients survive beyond 7 yrs
- Transplantations secondary to emphysema (mostly SLT) and cystic fibrosis (DLT) carry the best survival
- Transplantations secondary to pulmonary hypertension carry the worst survival
- Complications are frequent and may be fatal
- Early death (<90 days post-op) most commonly occurs from infection, donor organ failure, rejection, hemorrhage, or airway dehiscence
- Late death most commonly occurs from infection, chronic rejection/obliterative bronchiolitis, respiratory failure, or malignancy
- Obliterative bronchiolitis is an irreversible inflammatory disorder of the small airways that occurs in 50% of long-term lung transplant recipients and results in respiratory failure

Cardiac Surgery

Section 13

WALTER E. McGREGOR, MD

118. Cardiac Anatomy, Facts, and Pearls

- The heart can be affected by coronary atherosclerotic disease (the leading cause of mortality in developed countries), valve disease, rhythm disturbances, cardiac tumors, and progressive deterioration in heart function (chronic heart failure)
- Four cardiac chambers: Right atrium (RA), right ventricle (RV), left atrium (LA), left ventricle (LV)
- Normal blood flow pattern: Venous return from superior and inferior venae cavae and coronary sinus to the RA → tricuspid valve → RV → pulmonic valve → pulmonary arteries → to the lungs for oxygenation and gas exchange → return to the heart via the four pulmonary veins → LA → mitral valve → LV → aortic valve → to aorta, coronary arteries, and systemic circulation

Tricuspid Valve
- Composed of three leaflets (septal, anterior, and posterior) named for their orientation to the interventricular septum
- Associated with three papillary muscles, which originate in the right ventricle and connect to the valve leaflets via the chordae tendinae
- The septal leaflet attaches near the interventricular septum, AV node, and Bundle of His; hence, injury to the conduction system, septum, or mitral valve may occur

Pulmonic Valve
- Composed of three leaflets (right, left, and anterior) named for their orientation to the aortic valve
- Pathology is most commonly due to congenital abnormalities, rather than adult disease

Mitral Valve
- Composed of two leaflets (septal/anterior leaflet, mural/posterior leaflet) named for their adjacent structures
- Associated with two papillary muscles, which originate in the left ventricle and connect to the valve leaflets via the chordae tendineae
- The anterior leaflet is intimately associated with portions of the aortic valve; thus, injury to the aortic valve can occur as a complication during mitral valve surgery
- Injury to the Bundle of His, circumflex coronary artery, or coronary sinus may occur as a complication during mitral valve surgery

Aortic Valve
- Composed of three cusps (left, right, and non-coronary cusps) named for their orientation to the coronary arteries
- Other valves, the interventricular septum, and the conduction system may be injured during aortic valve surgery

Coronary Arteries
- Three major coronary arteries supply the heart: Left anterior descending coronary artery (LAD), circumflex coronary artery (Cx), and right coronary artery (RCA)
- Left main trunk (LMT) divides into the LAD and Cx
- LAD gives off perpendicular branches to the anterior two-thirds of the interventricular septum (septal perforators) and branches onto the anterolateral wall of the left ventricle (diagonal branches)
- Cx produces branches that supply the lateral wall of the left ventricle (obtuse marginal branches); in 10–15% of the population, the Cx terminates as the left posterior descending coronary artery supplying the posterior one-third of the interventricular septum (termed "left dominant")
- RCA produces branches that supply the anterior wall of the right ventricle (acute marginal branches); in 80–85% of the population, the RCA terminates as the right posterior descending coronary artery supplying the posterior one-third of the interventricular septum (termed "right dominant")
- Blood supply to the SA node may arise from either the left or right coronary arteries
- Blood supply to the AV node is based on the origin of the PDA (85% left dominant, 10–15% right dominant)

Cardiopulmonary Bypass
- Purpose: Permits the heart and lungs to be excluded from the circulation while allowing deoxygenated venous blood to bypass the heart and lungs; systemic arterial circulation returns in an oxygenated state and with adequate perfusion pressure to support end-organ function; this allows the heart to be stopped and opened without risk of air embolism or blood obscuring the surgical field
- Pathophysiology: Exposure of blood to foreign substances causes activation of platelets, the intrinsic and extrinsic coagulation system, the fibrinolytic system, the compliment cascade, and the kallikrein-kinin system, which can result in thrombosis, consumption of coagulation factors, excessive fibrinolysis, and a systemic inflammatory response; large doses of heparin (300U/Kg) should be administered to limit contact activation of the coagulation, compliment, and kinin systems; anti-fibrinolytic medications (e.g., ε-aminocaproic acid or aprotinin) should be administered to limit activation of the fibrinolytic system
- Components:
  - Venous line: Drains venous blood from the patient into a venous reservoir
  - Cardiotomy suction: Removes spilled blood from the operative field into a venous reservoir
  - Vent: Removes blood from the cardiac chambers into a venous reservoir in order to keep the operative field clear, prevent ventricular distension, and prevent cardiac rewarming
  - Venous reservoir: A transient storage area for blood from the above sources, which can then be delivered to the pump
  - Biomedicus pump: Centrifugal pump that causes less trauma to blood elements than roller pumps; pumps blood through the remainder of the heart-lung machine and back to the patient to sustain adequate perfusion pressure
  - Heater/cooler: Changes the temperature of the blood to allow active cooling or warming of the patient
  - Membrane oxygenator: Allows gas exchange to maintain physiologic pO_2, pCO_2, and pH in blood returning to patient
  - Filter: A safety screen to remove gaseous or particulate matter from blood prior to its return to the arterial circulation
  - Cardioplegia solution: A high dose KCl solution used to arrest the heart, thereby allowing the surgeon to operate on a non-moving organ; also provides a metabolic substrate to prevent myocardial edema and buffer the pH of the myocardium

119. Coronary Artery Disease

Etiology/Pathophysiology

- Coronary artery disease is the coronary manifestation of systemic atherosclerosis
- Response to injury hypothesis: Flow abnormalities or other intimal injury results in accumulation of lipid laden macrophages (foam cells); these cells orchestrate smooth muscle cell proliferation and platelet aggregation, resulting in a fibrointimal cap that narrows the lumen of the vessel
- Over time, the fibrous cap can rupture and heal, resulting in progressive lumen narrowing (stenosis), or can rupture with massive platelet aggregation and clot formation, resulting in vessel thrombosis (occlusion)
- Angina results from coronary artery stenosis that limits myocardial blood flow to the point that myocardial oxygen demand exceeds myocardial oxygen supply
- Myocardial infarction results from coronary artery thrombosis, which severely limits myocardial blood flow and oxygen supply, leading to cardiac muscle necrosis
- Risk factors for CAD include family history, diabetes mellitus, obesity, hypercholesterolemia, smoking, and hypertension

Differential Dx

- All causes of chest pain, arm pain, neck pain
  - Angina
  - Myocardial infarction
  - Pericarditis
  - Aortic dissection
  - Pneumothorax
  - Pulmonary embolus
  - Pleurisy
  - Pancoast tumor
  - Esophageal reflux/motility disorders
  - Peptic ulcer disease

Presentation/Signs & Symptoms

- Substernal, crushing chest pain with radiation to the left arm and jaw is the classic presentation
- Dyspnea on exertion
- Exercise limitation
- Nausea
- Bradycardia
- "Silent" (asymptomatic) disease may occur; more common in diabetics (due to neuropathy of visceral sensory pain fibers) and elderly patients

Diagnostic Evaluation

- ECG, chest X-ray, arterial blood gas, cardiac enzymes (e.g., CK-MB, troponins) are indicated to evaluate the acuity of myocardial insult
- Stress testing will confirm the presence of myocardial ischemia in patients who do not have clear evidence of infarction/necrosis
  - Treadmill stress testing if able to ambulate
  - Pharmacologic stress testing with adenosine or dobutamine if patient cannot undergo treadmill testing
- Echocardiogram will evaluate for accompanying valvular disease and cardiac function
- Cardiac catheterization with coronary angiography is indicated if there is a high clinical suspicion of CAD (e.g., suspicious history and physical exam, positive family history, positive cardiac enzymes, positive stress testing) to determine how many coronary arteries are blocked and the degree and location of the blockages

Treatment/Management

- Treatment options include medical treatment, angioplasty with stenting, or surgical revascularization
  - Medical treatment (e.g., aspirin, nitrates, β-blockers) may be used for patients with angina or mild disease, and those who do not proceed to cardiac catheterization
  - Angioplasty with stenting is indicated for patients with >50–70% stenosis
  - Surgical revascularization (i.e., coronary artery bypass grafting or CABG) provides a survival advantage over other options in patients with poor left ventricular function

Prognosis/Complications

- Complications following CABG or any open-heart surgery include bleeding, mediastinitis, stroke, respiratory failure, renal failure, and MI
- 2–5% operative mortality following CABG
- 85–90% 5-year survival following CABG
- Patients undergoing CABG require fewer follow-up interventions to maintain vessel patency than patients receiving angioplasty

120. Aortic Stenosis

Etiology/Pathophysiology

- Aortic stenosis (AS) results from any process that narrows the aortic valve aperture, thereby decreasing the aortic valve surface area (AVSA)
  - Progressive valvular "wear and tear" or other alterations in the normal valve anatomy result in valvular calcification, non-pliable valve cusps, and a decrease in AVSA
  - The left ventricle must generate greater systolic pressure in order to pump blood past the stenotic aortic valve to the rest of the body; this causes elevated left ventricular afterload and increased myocardial oxygen requirements
  - This systolic overload results in concentric hypertrophy of the left ventricle—the increased ventricular thickness leads to poor diastolic perfusion of the subendocardial myocardium, ischemia, dysfunction of myocytes, and heart failure
- Etiologies include a congenital bicuspid aortic valve (most common cause), senile calcific aortic stenosis (most common in ages >70 years), and rheumatic valve disease

Differential Dx

- Other causes of chest pain, dyspnea, and syncope
- Coronary artery disease
- Ischemic cardiomyopathy
- Idiopathic cardiomyopathy
- Hypertrophic cardiomyopathy (IHSS)
- Bilateral carotid stenosis

Presentation/Signs & Symptoms

- Angina
- Symptoms of heart failure (e.g., exercise intolerance, dyspnea on exertion, SOB) occur due to pulmonary edema, which is induced by the hypertrophied, noncompliant left ventricle
- Syncope secondary to myocyte dysfunction and ventricular arrhythmias
- May rarely be asymptomatic; however, upon careful questioning, patients usually will admit to limitations in exercise capacity
- Harsh, blowing systolic ejection murmur, greatest at the right second intercostal space
- Atrial fibrillation may ultimately occur with any untreated valvular pathology

Diagnostic Evaluation

- History and physical examination
- ECG and chest X-ray will show evidence of LV hypertrophy and will rule out other differentials
- Echocardiogram will evaluate for LV hypertrophy, decreased AVSA (normal is 2.5–3.5 cm^2), and an increased gradient across aortic valve
- If surgery is being considered, cardiac catheterization is indicated to directly measure AVSA, left ventricular end-diastolic pressure, and pulmonary artery pressure and evaluate for synchronous coronary artery disease

Treatment/Management

- Blood pressure reduction with a β-blocker is first-line therapy
- Surgical aortic valve replacement is indicated for symptomatic patients with severe aortic stenosis (AVSA <0.8 cm^2 or mean gradient >50 mmHg)
  - Bioprosthetic valves (porcine valve or bovine pericardial valve) have a lower risk of thromboembolic events and do not require long-term anticoagulation; however, they last only 10–15 years (usually adequate for patients >65 years)
  - Mechanical valves result in a greater risk of thromboembolic events, necessitating long-term anticoagulation; on the positive side, these valves will usually last for the life of the patient
- For asymptomatic patients with severe aortic stenosis, surgery is recommended if symptoms occur during stress testing or if high blood flow velocities are demonstrated across the aortic valve

Prognosis/Complications

- Prognosis of AS is poor without surgery
  - 1–2-year median survival for patients who present with heart failure
  - 3-year median survival for patients who present with syncope
  - 5-year median survival for patients who present with angina
- Surgical mortality is usually <5%
- 85% 5-year survival after valve replacement
- Complications include prosthetic valve endocarditis (SBE prophylaxis is recommended for all patients following any valve replacement), stroke/thromboembolic event (1–2% per year), anticoagulant associated bleeding (2–4% per year), valve thrombosis (<1% per year), and structural valve degeneration (bioprosthetic, 30% at 10 years; mechanical, 0% at 10 years)

121. Aortic Insufficiency

Etiology/Pathophysiology

- Aortic insufficiency (AI) results from pathologic processes that alter the aortic valve cusps or the anatomic structures to which the cusps attach (the aorta and aortic annulus)
  - Aortic pathologies may include an ascending aortic aneurysm, syphilitic aneurysm, or aortic dissection
  - Annulus pathologies include aorto-annular ectasia associated with connective tissue diseases (Marfan's or Ehlers-Danlos syndrome)
  - Valve cusp pathologies include myxomatous degeneration, rheumatic valve disease, endocarditis (which can also invade the annulus), or congenital bicuspid valve
- The pathophysiology of any valvular insufficiency is volume overload:
  - Increased left ventricular end-diastolic volume leads to progressive LV dilatation with eccentric hypertrophy
  - The increasing LV radius with decreased wall thickness results in increased wall stress and a decline in systolic function
  - Ultimately, congestive heart failure occurs

Differential Dx

- Other causes of dyspnea and CHF
  - Cardiac disease (e.g., acute MI, ischemic cardiomyopathy, idiopathic cardiomyopathy)
  - Pulmonary disease (e.g., COPD, interstitial lung disease)

Presentation/Signs & Symptoms

- Patients present with varying degrees of heart failure as left ventricular function worsens (e.g., exercise intolerance, dyspnea on exertion, fulminant CHF)
- Diastolic decrescendo murmur along the left sternal border
- Widened pulse pressure
- Atrial fibrillation may ultimately occur with any untreated valvular pathology

Diagnostic Evaluation

- Severity of heart failure is classified based on the New York Heart Association (NYHA) classification
  - Class I: No symptoms with physical activity
  - Class II: Symptoms with normal activity
  - Class III: Symptoms with less than normal activity
  - Class IV: Symptoms at rest
- ECG and CXR are used to evaluate cardiac enlargement and rule out other diseases (e.g., acute MI, COPD)
- Echocardiogram will evaluate the degree of regurgitant flow, valve and aortic pathology, end-diastolic and end-systolic dimensions, systolic function (i.e., ejection fraction), and synchronous valvular disease (e.g., mitral regurgitation)
- If surgical intervention is planned, cardiac catheterization is indicated to determine the cardiac chamber pressures and evaluate for synchronous coronary artery disease

Treatment/Management

- Blood pressure reduction with an ACE inhibitor is first-line therapy
- Surgical intervention is indicated once a decline in systolic cardiac function occurs (e.g., presence of CHF symptoms, decreased ejection fraction, poor systolic response to exercise testing, dilated end-systolic diameter)
- Surgery is directed toward the underlying pathology, and may include aortic valve replacement, ascending aorta replacement, or (rarely) aortic valve repair
  - Bioprosthetic valves (porcine valve or bovine pericardial valve) have a lower risk of thromboembolic events and do not require long-term anticoagulation; however, they last only 10–15 years (usually adequate for patients >65 years)
  - Mechanical valves result in a greater risk of thromboembolic events, necessitating long-term anticoagulation; on the positive side, these valves will usually last for the life of the patient

Prognosis/Complications

- Prognosis depends on the degree of ventricular dysfunction and severity of heart failure
  - 50% 1-year survival for class IV patients
  - 70% 1-year survival for class III patients
- Surgical mortality and 5-year survival after valve replacement for AI is 5–10% and 60–90%, respectively, depending on the degree of LV dysfunction
- Complications include prosthetic valve endocarditis (SBE prophylaxis is recommended for all patients following any valve replacement), stroke/thromboembolic events (1–2% per year), anticoagulant-associated bleeding (2–4% per year), valve thrombosis (<1% per year), and structural valve degeneration (bioprosthetic, 30% at 10 years; mechanical, 0% at 10 years)

122. Mitral Stenosis

Etiology/Pathophysiology

- Mitral stenosis (MS) almost always results from rheumatic heart disease; however, a history of rheumatic fever is present in only 50% of cases
- The stenotic mitral valve protects the left ventricle (LV) and preserves left ventricular function, but limits LV filling leading to a diminished cardiac output and blood stasis in the left atrium
    - Limited LV filling results in CHF and decreased cardiac output
    - Blood stasis in the left atrium results in atrial fibrillation and pulmonary edema

Differential Dx

- Other causes of dyspnea and CHF
    - Cardiac disease (e.g., acute MI, ischemic cardiomyopathy, idiopathic cardiomyopathy)
    - Pulmonary disease (e.g., COPD, interstitial lung disease)

Presentation/Signs & Symptoms

- Atrial fibrillation is often the presenting sign of mitral stenosis
- Symptoms of heart failure (e.g., exercise intolerance, dyspnea on exertion, fulminant CHF)
- Auscultatory triad is often heard
    - Increased first heart sound
    - Opening snap
    - Diastolic rumble
- Hemoptysis occurs secondary to pulmonary edema

Diagnostic Evaluation

- History and physical examination
- ECG and chest X-ray will evaluate for atrial fibrillation and rule out other causes of CHF
- Echocardiogram is used to evaluate valve pathology, degree of stenosis (normal mitral valve surface area is 4–6 cm^2), extent of rheumatic involvement (e.g., valve leaflets, subvalvular apparatus, depressed LV function), left atrial enlargement, presence of clots in the left atrium, and synchronous valve disease from rheumatic fever
- If surgery is planned, cardiac catheterization is indicated to evaluate cardiac chamber pressures, pulmonary artery hypertension, MVSA, and synchronous coronary artery disease

Treatment/Management

- Surgical treatment is indicated once patients become symptomatic or develops atrial fibrillation, an enlarged left atrium (>4–5 cm), or a highly stenotic valve (MVSA <1.0 cm^2)
    - Balloon valvuloplasty may be used for mild disease
    - Open mitral commissurotomy is indicated for more extensive disease (e.g., leaflet fusion, tethering of the chordae tendineae of the subvalvular apparatus)
    - Mitral valve replacement is indicated when commissurotomy is prohibitive or fails (valve options are detailed in the "Aortic Insufficiency" entry)

Prognosis/Complications

- In addition to the generic risks of valve replacement (see "Aortic Insufficiency" entry), additional risks of mitral valve replacement include atrioventricular groove dissociation (large hole in posterior aspect of heart)
- Complications are lowered following mitral valve repair versus replacement
- 5% operative mortality following mitral valve replacement
- 80% 5-year survival following mitral valve replacement

123. Mitral Insufficiency

Etiology/Pathophysiology

- Mitral regurgitation (MR) results from pathologic changes of the mitral leaflets or the structures to which they attach (mitral annulus, chordae tendineae, papillary muscles, or left ventricle)
- Etiologies include myxomatous degeneration (most common cause), rheumatic valve disease, endocarditis, and ischemia (acute or chronic)
  - Acute ischemic MR may be secondary to an infarcted and ruptured papillary muscle or ventricular wall/papillary muscle dysfunction related to an acute MI or severe ischemia
  - Chronic ischemic MR results from long-term dysfunction of the left ventricle due to chronic ischemia or prior MIs with remodeling of normal ventricular geometry
- The pathophysiology of any valvular insufficiency is volume overload:
  - Increased left ventricular end-diastolic volume leads to progressive LV dilatation with eccentric hypertrophy
  - The increasing LV radius with decreased wall thickness results in increased wall stress and a decline in systolic function
  - Ultimately, congestive heart failure occurs

Differential Dx

- Other causes of dyspnea and CHF
  - Cardiac disease (e.g., acute MI, ischemic cardiomyopathy, idiopathic cardiomyopathy)
  - Pulmonary disease (e.g., COPD, interstitial lung disease)

Presentation/Signs & Symptoms

- Patients present with varying degrees of heart failure as left ventricular function worsens (e.g., exercise intolerance, dyspnea on exertion, fulminant CHF)
- Apical systolic murmur radiating to the axilla
- Atrial fibrillation may ultimately occur with any untreated valvular pathology

Diagnostic Evaluation

- History and physical examination
- Severity of heart failure is graded based on the New York Heart Association (NYHA) classification
  - Class I: No symptoms with physical activity
  - Class II: Symptoms with normal activity
  - Class III: Symptoms with less than normal activity
  - Class IV: Symptoms at rest
- ECG and chest X-ray are used to evaluate cardiac enlargement and rule out other disease processes
- Echocardiogram will define the degree of regurgitation and underlying pathologic mechanism
- If surgery is planned, cardiac catheterization is indicated to determine cardiac chamber pressures, pulmonary artery pressures, and evaluate for synchronous coronary artery disease

Treatment/Management

- Blood pressure reduction with an ACE inhibitor is first-line therapy
- Surgical intervention is indicated once a decline in systolic cardiac function occurs (e.g., presence of CHF symptoms, decreased ejection fraction, poor systolic response to exercise testing, dilated end-systolic diameter)
- Surgery (mitral valve repair or replacement) should be directed toward the underlying pathology
  - MV repair is preferable (most successful in cases of myxomatous valve degeneration); however, if the mechanism of MR is not clear, the valve should be replaced rather than repaired
  - See "Aortic Insufficiency" entry for valve replacement options

Prognosis/Complications

- In addition to the generic risks of valve replacement (see "Aortic Insufficiency" entry), additional risks of mitral valve replacement include atrioventricular groove dissociation (large hole in posterior aspect of heart)
- Risks are lowered for valve repair versus replacement
- 5% operative mortality following isolated mitral valve replacement
- 80% 5-year survival after isolated mitral valve replacement

124. Left Ventricular Aneurysm

Etiology/Pathophysiology

- Left ventricular aneurysms (LVA) result from transmural infarction of the left anterior descending (resulting in an anterior aneurysm) or posterior descending (resulting in a posterior aneurysm) coronary arteries
    - One-third of patients have coronary artery disease (CAD) isolated to the left anterior descending (LAD) artery territory
    - Two-thirds of patients have multivessel CAD
- Over weeks to months, transmural infarction leads to scar formation, thinning of the ventricular wall, and eventual asymmetric enlargement of the LV cavity with dyskinetic (paradoxic) wall motion in the aneurysmal area
- This pathologic remodeling of the LV cavity leads to an increase in wall stress, which leads to an increase in myocardial oxygen consumption and eventual deterioration of ventricular function
- Posterior LVA can distort the mitral valve, resulting in mitral regurgitation
- Pseudoaneurysm should be differentiated from true aneurysm formation
    - Pseudoaneurysm results from acute transmural infarction leading to ventricular free wall rupture and containment by the pericardium
    - These have an unstable natural history and should be repaired regardless of symptoms or size

Differential Dx

- Ventricular pseudoaneurysm
- Ventricular dilation with scar formation but only an akinetic scar segment (no paradoxic motion)

Presentation/Signs & Symptoms

- Angina due to coexisting coronary occlusive disease
- Symptoms of CHF (e.g., exercise intolerance, dyspnea on exertion, SOB)
    - Aneurysms <5 cm in diameter rarely cause heart failure symptoms
- Ventricular arrhythmias may result from arrhythmogenic foci around the base of the dyskinetic scar segment
- Peripheral emboli may result from systemic embolization of mural thrombi that occur due to stagnant blood flow within the left ventricular aneurysm

Diagnostic Evaluation

- History and physical exam
- ECG and chest X-ray evaluate for other pathology
- Echocardiogram evaluates LVA anatomy and size, presence of mural thrombi, LV function, and associated valvular dysfunction
- Electrophysiologic mapping is indicated if there is a history of arrhythmias in order to facilitate resection of the arrhythmogenic foci during the surgical repair of the LVA
- If surgical intervention is planned, cardiac catheterization is indicated to evaluate cardiac chamber pressures and extent of coronary occlusive disease

Treatment/Management

- Surgical repair is indicated for all symptomatic cases
- The classic repair involves resection of the aneurysm, removal of thrombi, and linear closure of scar rim using Teflon felt strips
    - Closure of large aneurysms may distort and undersize the left ventricle
- Ventricular reconstructive aneurysm repairs may involve Dacron or pericardial patches to close the resulting ventricular defect and minimize undersizing of the LV
- Coronary revascularization should be performed whenever possible

Prognosis/Complications

- 50% 5-year survival without surgery
- 60–80% 5-year survival with surgery
- 4–8% operative mortality

125. Acute (Post-Infarct) Ventricular Septal Defect

Etiology/Pathophysiology

- Acute ventricular septal defect (VSD) is a surgical emergency caused by an acute myocardial infarction involving the left anterior descending (LAD) or posterior descending (PDA) coronary arteries
    - Acute occlusion of either artery leads to transmural necrosis of the interventricular septum, tissue loss, and a resulting hole in the interventricular septum
    - Acute occlusion of the LAD results in an anterior VSD (i.e., the anterior portion of the interventricular septum is damaged)
    - Acute occlusion of the PDA results in a posterior VSD (i.e., the posterior portion of the interventricular septum is damaged)
- The acute formation of a VSD results in a left-to-right shunt, leading to acute volume overload of the right ventricle and pulmonary vasculature, and ultimately right ventricular dysfunction and congestive heart failure with low cardiac output

Differential Dx

- Post-infarct mitral regurgitation due to a ruptured/torn papillary muscle
- Post-infarct ventricular free wall rupture with cardiac tamponade
- Extension of myocardial infarct with massive loss of myocardial tissue and resultant CHF

Presentation/Signs & Symptoms

- Onset of CHF and low cardiac output following an acute myocardial infarction (typically occurs within the first week following an acute MI)
    - Symptoms of pulmonary edema (e.g., dyspnea, rales)
    - Cool, underperfused extremities
    - Diminished urine output
- Holosystolic murmur

Diagnostic Evaluation

- ECG and cardiac enzymes will reveal an acute MI
- Chest X-ray will reveal pulmonary edema
- Pulmonary artery catheterization will diagnose the left-to-right shunt
    - Normally, blood oxygen saturation is low throughout the entire right heart
    - With left-to-right shunting, blood oxygen saturation increases in the right heart
    - Increase in blood oxygen saturation is detected by sampling blood from the right atrium (drawn from the central venous line) versus blood from the pulmonary artery (drawn from a pulmonary artery catheter)
- Echocardiogram demonstrates the left-to-right shunt, anatomy of the defect, and underlying LV function
- Cardiac catheterization is used to diagnose and evaluate the degree of left-to-right shunt and evaluate the extent of coronary occlusive disease

Treatment/Management

- Initial management entails stabilization of cardiopulmonary status with an intra-aortic balloon pump and, if needed, mechanical ventilation
- Early surgical closure of the VSD is required in most cases; some patients with minimal symptoms will benefit from a delayed closure (2–3 weeks) to allow the infarcted tissue time to develop scar in order to hold sutures more securely

Prognosis/Complications

- Complications include recurrent VSD due to breakdown of the suture line (related to the quality of the tissue and friability of the recent infarct)
- Operative mortality for an anterior VSD is 15%
- Operative mortality for a posterior VSD is 30%
- Mortality increases in the presence of cardiogenic shock
- 5-year survival is 70%, but is dependent on the degree of LV dysfunction

126. Heart Transplantation

Etiology/Pathophysiology

- Cardiac transplantation is considered for end-stage heart failure when medical, percutaneous, and surgical treatments are no longer successful or are not an option
- The most common indications for heart transplant are idiopathic dilated cardiomyopathy and ischemic cardiomyopathy
- Cardiac transplantation is typically offered only to patients who satisfy specific criteria
  - End-stage heart disease in a young person (<55–65 years of age)
  - Limited evidence of end-organ dysfunction
  - No other good treatment options
  - Absence of active infection or malignancy
  - Poor predictors of 1-year survival
  - No evidence of fixed pulmonary hypertension, since the normal donor heart right ventricle is not accustomed to pumping against high pulmonary resistance, placing the donor heart into a recipient with a high pulmonary resistance will result in right ventricular failure, allograft failure, and recipient death

Differential Dx

Presentation/Signs & Symptoms

- Absolute contraindications to transplant include active infection, persistent malignancy, irreversible pulmonary hypertension, pulmonary vascular resistance >6 woods units, and transpulmonary gradient (mean pulmonary artery pressure – pulmonary capillary wedge pressure) >15 mmHg
- Predictors of poor survival without transplant
  - NYHA class IV symptoms (50% 1-year survival at best)
  - NYHA class III symptoms (70% 1-year survival at best)
  - Ejection fraction <20%
  - Exercise testing with low vO_2 max
  - Home dobutamine infusion

Diagnostic Evaluation

- History and physical exam
- ECG and chest X-ray
- Laboratory studies: Evaluate viral titers, end-organ dysfunction, and evidence of occult malignancy
- Echocardiogram should be used to evaluate myocardial geometry and function and presence of valvular disease
- Myocardial viability study evaluates the myocardium for potential for improvement with revascularization
- Cardiac catheterization will evaluate pulmonary artery pressures and pulmonary vascular resistance, LV function, coronary occlusive disease, and quality of coronary arteries for bypass grafting
- Exercise testing to evaluate vO_2 max

Treatment/Management

- Two surgical options: Atrial cuff anastomosis versus bicaval anastomosis
  - Atrial cuff anastomosis is an easier operation: Diseased heart is removed with the exception of a cuff of right and left atrium; donor heart is then anastomosed by sewing left atrium to left atrial cuff, right atrium to right atrial cuff
  - Bicaval anastomosis results in fewer cases of postoperative arrhythmias and valve insufficiency: Diseased heart is removed entirely; the donor heart is then anastomosed by sewing donor SVC to SVC and donor IVC to IVC

Prognosis/Complications

- 80% 1-year, 65% 5-year, and 35% 12-year survival
- Postoperative complications
  - Cardiac dysfunction (e.g., due to prolonged ischemia during transport of donor heart)
  - Hyperacute rejection (minutes to hours) mediated by preformed antibodies
  - Acute rejection (weeks to months) mediated by activated T-cells that recognize non-self MHC antigens on donor cells
  - Chronic rejection (years) mediated by humoral and cellular mechanisms resulting in graft atherosclerosis
  - Infection: May be bacterial (pneumonia), viral (CMV), fungal (candidiasis), or parasitic (PCP)
  - Post-transplant lymphoproliferative disorder: B-cell lymphoma related to chronic EBV infection

Neurosurgery

JACK E. WILBERGER, MD, FACS

Section 14

127. Intracranial Aneurysms

Etiology/Pathophysiology

- Intracranial aneurysms are present in up to 10% of the population and become symptomatic at the rate of 7.5/100,000/year
- Most aneurysms are congenital, caused by abnormalities in the arterial wall; a small number of cases occur post-traumatically or secondary to infection (mycotic aneurysms)
- Rupture of an aneurysm generally results in a subarachnoid hemorrhage (SAH)—80% of cases of SAH are due to rupture of an intracranial aneurysm (trauma is the next most common cause of SAH)
  - Aneurysm rupture resulting in SAH is most likely beyond age 40
  - Paradoxically, smaller aneurysms (<2 cm) are more likely to rupture than larger aneurysms
  - The mortality from aneurysm rupture is as high as 33%, with an additional 33% mortality or severe neurologic impairment secondary to complications (e.g., cerebral vasospasm)
- There is a 20% risk of acute re-hemorrhage during the initial 2 weeks following an untreated ruptured aneurysm; after 6 months the risk drops to 1–2%/year
- Asymptomatic aneurysms found incidentally have a 1–2%/year risk of eventual rupture

Differential Dx

- With presence of SAH
  - Arteriovenous malformation
  - Trauma
  - Brain tumor
- Without SAH
  - Brain tumor
  - Seizure disorder
  - Drug intoxication
  - Metabolic disturbance

Presentation/Signs & Symptoms

- Pressure of the aneurysm on surrounding structures may result in focal neurologic deficits (e.g., third cranial nerve palsy with a dilated ipsilateral pupil, brainstem dysfunction)
- Patients with ruptured aneurysm will present with signs of SAH
  - Severe headache ("worst headache of my life")
  - Irritability
  - Altered mental status
  - Photophobia
  - Nausea/vomiting
  - Meningismus
  - Syncope and/or seizures may occur
  - Coma

Diagnostic Evaluation

- CT scan without contrast is generally the initial test-of-choice to reveal subarachnoid or intraventricular hemorrhage; however, the aneurysm itself will rarely be visualized (though large aneurysms may be seen)
  - SAH will be visible in the basal cisterns, sylvian fissure, interhemispheric space, and posterior fossa
- Lumbar puncture may be done if CT is negative
  - SAH will be positive for xanthochromia or elevated RBCs, which do not clear with continued fluid collection
- Cerebral angiography is the gold standard to delineate the aneurysm; however, only used if the diagnosis is in doubt
- Angiography with MR (MRA) or CT (CTA) may also be used
- Rule out other possible causes of intracerebral hemorrhage
  - PT/PTT/INR to rule out clotting disorders
  - Toxicology screen to rule out cocaine abuse
  - CBC to rule out thrombocytopenia

Treatment/Management

- Blood pressure stabilization and control to prevent re-bleeding
- Prevent/ameliorate vasospasm
  - Nimodipine (calcium channel blocker) administration is indicated in all patients unless significant hypotension occurs; administer every 6 hours for 21 days
  - Hypertension, hypervolemia, and hemodilution ("Triple-H" therapy)
- Ventricular CSF drainage to decrease ICP if hydrocephalus is present on CT scan
- Surgery (preferably within 24–48 hours from SAH) is indicated to secure the aneurysm and prevent re-bleeding in medically stable patients
- Angiography with selective embolization and clipping may be indicated
- Seizure prophylaxis in some patients

Prognosis/Complications

- Vasospasm of cerebral vessels is a feared consequence
  - Irritation of vessels by blood breakdown products results in ischemia or infarction
  - Occurs in up to 30% of cases
  - Peak incidence 3–7 days after SAH
- Hyponatremia (due to cerebral salt wasting syndrome) commonly occurs
- Hydrocephalus following SAH may cause delayed recovery and/or new deficits
- Of patients who survive the initial SAH, >60% will have a good outcome
  - 10–15% will die from complications of the disease
  - 10% will be left severely disabled
  - 15% become mildly disabled

128. Epidural Hematoma

Etiology/Pathophysiology

- An uncommon result of closed head injuries; usually associated with a skull fracture
- Most common in 15–30 year old males following a motor vehicle crash; seen on occasion following falls or sporting activities
- Epidural bleeding most often occurs in the fronto-temporal regions secondary to damage of the middle meningeal artery or its branches, resulting in rapid neurologic signs and symptoms
    - Arterial bleeding leads to a rapid rise in intracranial pressure (ICP), followed by uncal herniation and brainstem compression
- Venous bleeding may occur secondary to venous sinus injuries or "venous lakes" in the dura, resulting in a relatively slow onset of neurologic signs/symptoms; common in the posterior fossa in children
- Secondary brain injury: Additional insults following injury (e.g., hypotension, hypoxia, brain swelling) may propagate further cerebral tissue damage by decreasing cerebral perfusion pressure

Differential Dx

- Intracranial mass lesion
    - Subdural hematoma
    - Intracerebral hematoma
    - Contusion
    - Tumor
- Seizure disorder
- Drug intoxication
- Metabolic coma
- Stroke
- Traumatic subarachnoid hemorrhage

Presentation/Signs & Symptoms

- History of head injury followed by a lucid interval (up to 60 minutes) and subsequent neurologic decline to coma
- Severe headache
- Seizures
- Vomiting (especially in children)
- Brainstem herniation is indicated by palsy of the third cranial nerve, usually resulting in ipsilateral pupil dilation, and contralateral hemiparesis

Diagnostic Evaluation

- History and physical exam, including detailed neurologic exam
- Head CT without contrast
    - Findings include convex hyperdensity, shift of midline structures, compression of ipsilateral ventricles, and dilation of contralateral ventricles
- C-spine films may be indicated to rule out associated cervical injury

Treatment/Management

- Maintain airway, breathing, and circulation
- Seizure prophylaxis in all patients (e.g., phenytoin)
- Surgical evacuation with control of bleeding source
- Begin intracranial pressure monitoring (i.e., via ventricular catheter or fiber optic monitor) if consciousness is not rapidly regained
- Prevent/ameliorate secondary brain injury
    - IV fluid administration to prevent hypotension
    - Intubation for hypoxia
    - Mannitol or furosemide administration to relieve cerebral edema
    - Relieve elevated intracranial pressure by head elevation, mild hyperventilation (e.g., pCO_2=35), mannitol and/or furosemide administration, and surgical drainage
- Burr-hole evacuation if no other treatment is available

Prognosis/Complications

- Excellent outcome if treated early
- Rarely associated with other significant intracranial injuries
- 20% mortality
- Sudden death may occur

129. Subdural Hematoma

Etiology/Pathophysiology

- Acute subdural hematoma occurs in association with severe closed head injury
  - The most common and most lethal of post-traumatic intracranial lesions
  - Typically due to shearing of cortical veins with significant associated brain injury
  - Commonly associated with parenchymal brain lesions, such as contusions, hematoma, and diffuse axonal injury
  - Increased frequency in the elderly, especially those on anticoagulation
- Chronic subdural hematoma presents 1–2 months after a usually trivial, and often unremembered, head trauma
  - Initially, small amounts of subdural blood accumulate
  - Progressive enlargement occurs due to defects in local fibrinolytic pathways or use of anticoagulation
- Secondary brain injury: Additional insults following injury (e.g., hypotension, hypoxia, brain swelling) may propagate further cerebral tissue damage by decreasing cerebral perfusion pressure

Differential Dx

- Acute subdural hematoma
  - Intracranial mass lesion (e.g., epidural hematoma, intracerebral hematoma)
  - Spontaneous intracerebral hematoma (e.g., hypertensive)
  - Seizure disorder
  - Drug intoxication
  - Metabolic coma
- Chronic subdural
  - Dementia
  - Intracranial mass lesion
  - Seizure disorder
  - Drug intoxication
  - Metabolic disturbances

Presentation/Signs & Symptoms

- Acute subdural hematoma
  - Patient typically presents in a coma soon after trauma
  - Progressive deterioration and deepening coma
  - Focal neurologic signs
- Chronic subdural hematoma
  - Slowly developing symptoms with gradual neurologic symptoms
  - Headaches
  - Drowsiness
  - Mental status changes
  - Dementia
  - Gait disturbance
  - Seizures
  - Focal neurologic signs

Diagnostic Evaluation

- History and physical exam, including a detailed neurologic examination
- Head CT without contrast will show a crescent-shaped, concave hyperdensity (in acute subdural) or hypodensity (in chronic subdural), cerebral edema, and contusions
- Head MRI is indicated if chronic subdural hematoma is suspected to distinguish from a hygroma (benign CSF collection)

Treatment/Management

- Airway, breathing, and circulation
- Seizure prophylaxis (e.g., phenytoin)
- Acute subdural hematoma
  - Surgical evacuation and control of bleeding is indicated if patient is neurologically salvageable
  - Intracranial pressure monitoring and treatment
  - Prevent/ameliorate secondary brain injuries (IV fluid administration to prevent hypotension; intubation to prevent hypoxia; relieve elevated intracranial pressure by head elevation, mild hyperventilation (e.g., pCO_2=35), mannitol and/or furosemide administration, and surgical drainage)
- Chronic subdural hematoma
  - If significant signs are not present, patients may be managed conservatively with monitoring of neurologic status and serial CT scans
  - Evacuation of hematoma with or without associated drainage of subdural space

Prognosis/Complications

- Acute subdural hematoma has a very poor prognosis
  - >80% mortality, usually due to underlying brain injury
  - Early surgical intervention (<4 hours from time of injury) may slightly improve outcome
  - Complications are usually related to the need for prolonged ventilation (e.g., pneumonia, ARDS, sepsis, multisystem organ failure)
- Chronic subdural hematoma generally has a good prognosis as long as significant focal neurologic signs or coma are not present
  - >80% of cases have a satisfactory outcome
  - The hematoma may reaccumulate or recur, requiring additional surgical interventions

130. Hydrocephalus

Etiology/Pathophysiology

- May occur due to overproduction of cerebrospinal fluid (CSF), inadequate reabsorption of CSF by the arachnoid villi, or blockage of the normal CSF circulation pathways
- CSF accumulation and progressive enlargement of the cerebral ventricles results in progressive brain dysfunction
- Communicating hydrocephalus: Inadequate reabsorption of CSF most commonly secondary to trauma, infection, or subarachnoid hemorrhage
- Non-communicating hydrocephalus: Obstruction of CSF circulation pathways by tumors or congenital abnormalities (e.g., aqueductal stenosis, Arnold-Chiari malformation), such that CSF cannot escape from within the brain to the basal cisterns

Differential Dx

- Intracranial mass lesion
- Glycogen/lipid storage diseases
- Dementia

Presentation/Signs & Symptoms

- Children
  - Enlarging head, bulging fontanelles
  - Developmental delays
  - Lethargy
  - Vomiting
- Adults
  - Headaches
  - Cognitive disturbances
  - Nausea/vomiting
  - Dementia
  - Gait disturbances
  - Bladder incontinence
  - Seizures
  - Focal neurologic deficits
  - Papilledema (late)

Diagnostic Evaluation

- History and physical exam, including detailed neurologic examination
- Head CT without contrast
- Head MRI is indicated if aqueductal stenosis or Arnold-Chiari malformation is suspected
- Radioisotope CSF study is indicated if suspect communicating hydrocephalus; will reveal abnormal CSF circulation

Treatment/Management

- Communicating hydrocephalus
  - Acetazolamide (carbonic anhydrase inhibitor) administration will decrease CSF production
  - Repeated lumbar punctures to evacuate excess CSF
  - Ventriculoperitoneal or lumboperitoneal shunt is indicated in about one-third of cases and is the definitive treatment
- Non-communicating hydrocephalus
  - Removal of obstructing mass lesion
  - Ventriculoperitoneal shunting is indicated in nearly all cases
  - Ventriculostomy of the third ventricle is helpful in 15% of cases

Prognosis/Complications

- Prognosis is generally good with early diagnosis and appropriate treatment
- Significant neurologic dysfunction (either directly due to hydrocephalus or due to associated inciting conditions) is rarely reversed, even with aggressive treatment
- Multiple potential complications are associated with shunting, including intracerebral or intraventricular hemorrhage, infection, shunt malfunction, and subdural hematoma (due to overdrainage of CSF)

131. Cerebral Abscess

Etiology/Pathophysiology

- Most cases are due to infection of the adjacent skull or sinus with subsequent spread through the meninges
- Less common causes include penetrating head injury, intracranial foreign bodies (e.g., bullet fragments from gunshot wounds), and hematogenous spread
- Post-craniotomy patients have a 1–2% risk of infection/abscess
- Increased risk in immunosuppressed or immunocompromised patients
  – Toxoplasma is the most common organism in these patients

Differential Dx

- Meningitis
- Encephalitis
- Intracranial mass lesion

Presentation/Signs & Symptoms

- Headache
- Lethargy
- Fever/chills
- Seizures
- Focal neurologic deficits (e.g., arm/leg weakness)
- Coma

Diagnostic Evaluation

- History and physical exam, including detailed neurologic examination
- CBC with differential will reveal leukocytosis
- Blood cultures
- Head CT with contrast will reveal a ring-enhancing lesion with extensive edema
- Head MRI with enhancement is primarily used in immunocompromised patients since multiple lesions may be present

Treatment/Management

- Administer appropriate IV antibiotics or antifungal agents for 4–6 weeks
- Seizure prophylaxis for all patients (e.g., phenytoin)
- Surgical debridement, drainage, and culture are indicated for a large abscess that results in a significant mass effect, an abscess associated with foreign bodies, or an abscess with an unknown source of infection

Prognosis/Complications

- Prognosis is excellent when early diagnosis and appropriate treatment are provided
- Significant neurologic deficits may not be reversible despite appropriate treatment
- Long-term seizure disorders may result

132. Benign Brain Tumors

Etiology/Pathophysiology

- The majority of benign brain tumors arise from de novo genetic mutations
- On occasion, benign tumors may occur in conjunction with familial syndromes (e.g., neurofibromatosis type 2)
- The most common benign tumors are meningioma and neurofibroma or schwannoma
- Symptoms usually develop slowly, secondary to compression of adjacent brain tissue and/or cranial nerves

Differential Dx

- Malignant brain tumor
- Hydrocephalus
- Brain abscess
- Primary seizure disorder

Presentation/Signs & Symptoms

- Headaches
- Seizures
- Cranial nerve deficits (e.g., diplopia, facial weakness)
- Focal neurologic signs (e.g., arm/leg weakness)

Diagnostic Evaluation

- History and physical exam with detailed neurologic examination
- Head CT with and without contrast will identify 80% of tumors
- Head MRI with and without enhancement will help to identify tumors that do not appear on CT (e.g., meningioma)
- Audiometry and visual field testing is indicated for tumors involving ear or eye structures
- Cerebral angiogram may be used for vascular tumors to identify and/or embolize vessels when anticipating surgery (i.e., to decrease bleeding during surgery)

Treatment/Management

- Asymptomatic or incidentally found benign tumors may be followed with serial CT/MRI and serial clinical examinations
- Immediate steroid administration may be used to decrease any tumor-associated cerebral edema
- Symptomatic tumors generally require surgical removal
- For large tumors, cerebral angiography with embolization of large feeding vessels may be a helpful adjunct to surgery
- For smaller, residual, or recurrent benign tumors, radiation therapy may be indicated

Prognosis/Complications

- Approximately 5–10% of benign tumors will recur following complete surgical removal; thus, yearly CT or MRI are required for at least 5 years
- Cranial nerve deficits or other focal neurologic deficits are not likely to resolve despite tumor removal
- There is a 2–5% incidence of new deficits associated with treatment
- Long-term seizure disorders may result

133. Malignant Brain Tumors

Etiology/Pathophysiology

- Metastatic tumors (especially from breast, lung, and prostate) are the most common malignant brain tumors
- The majority of primary malignant brain tumors arise from de novo genetic mutations
    - Glioblastoma multiforme is the most common primary brain tumor
- Primary malignant tumors are classified according to the World Health Organization (WHO) guidelines (higher grade implies poorer prognosis)
    - Grade I: Pilocytic astrocytoma
    - Grade II: Astrocytoma
    - Grade III: Anaplastic astrocytoma
    - Grade IV: Glioblastoma multiforme

Differential Dx

- Benign brain tumor
- Cerebral abscess
- Hydrocephalus
- Primary seizure disorder

Presentation/Signs & Symptoms

- Headaches
- Seizures
- Nausea/vomiting
- Lethargy
- Focal neurologic deficits (e.g., arm/leg weakness)
    - The more malignant the tumor, the more rapid the loss of neurologic function

Diagnostic Evaluation

- History and physical exam, including a detailed neurologic examination
- Head CT with and without contrast will identify most cases
- Head MRI with and without enhancement
- Metastatic workup to identify the primary tumor, if appropriate
    - CT of the thorax, abdomen, and pelvis
    - Prostate specific antigen measurement
    - Mammogram
    - Hematologic and bone marrow examination for lymphoma

Treatment/Management

- Steroids should be administered in all cases to decrease peritumoral edema
- Metastatic tumors
    - Surgical removal followed by fractionated radiation therapy (administered in divided doses to decrease side effects) is used if two or fewer lesions are present, the primary tumor is known, and there is no disseminated disease
    - Fractionated radiation alone is indicated if disseminated disease or >2 lesions are present
    - Excisional or stereotaxic biopsy are used to treat lesions with an unknown primary tumor
- Primary tumors
    - Stereotaxic biopsy and/or open excision when possible
    - Fractionated radiation therapy
    - Chemotherapy

Prognosis/Complications

- Outcome of metastatic tumors primarily depends on control of the primary disease
- Primary, malignant tumor survival depends on the grade of the tumor
    - Grade I: >20 years
    - Grade II: >10 years
    - Grade III: <5 years
    - Grade IV: <3 years
- Radiation therapy may be complicated by radiation necrosis of the surrounding brain tissue
    - Dementia occurs in 5% of cases
- Chemotherapy is often associated with systemic side effects

134. Spinal Cord Compression

Etiology/Pathophysiology

- A medical emergency that occurs when pressure on the spinal cord causes bilateral loss of motor and sensory function below the lesion
- Etiologies of spinal cord compression
    - Spinal column trauma (e.g., bone fragments, epidural hematoma, acute disc herniation)
    - Primary tumors (e.g., neurofibromas, meningiomas)
    - Metastatic tumors (e.g., breast cancer, prostate cancer)
    - Epidural abscess
    - Degenerative conditions (e.g., spondylosis, disc herniation)
- Ultimately, loss of adequate blood flow to neural tissue results in spinal cord dysfunction

Differential Dx

- Demyelinating diseases (e.g., multiple sclerosis)
- Motor neuron disease (e.g., amyotrophic lateral sclerosis)
- Autoimmune disorders (e.g., Guillain-Barré syndrome, transverse myelitis)
- Infections (e.g., polio, West Nile virus)

Presentation/Signs & Symptoms

- Spinal and/or radicular pain
- Numbness or tingling of extremities
- Acute or progressive loss of motor and sensory function
- Either incontinence or constipation may occur due to loss of sphincter control
- Symptoms and signs of the underlying process may be evident (e.g., fever in cases of infection, weight loss in cases of malignancy, signs of trauma)

Diagnostic Evaluation

- History and physical exam, including detailed neurologic examination
    - Give particular attention to upper and lower extremity muscle strength testing and dermatomal sensation
- Plain spine films are useful in cases of trauma or metastatic disease
- Spine MRI is the gold standard for diagnosing cord compression
- CT with myelogram is used in patients unable to undergo MRI (e.g., too large to fit in MRI machine, claustrophobia)

Treatment/Management

- Immediate steroid administration in all patients
    - IV methylprednisolone 30 mg/kg bolus plus 5.4 mg/kg/hr for 23 hours
- Treat underlying conditions as appropriate
    - Radiation therapy to treat metastatic disease, as long as the spinal column is stable
    - Craniocervical traction for post-traumatic cervical spine subluxation
    - IV antibiotics for epidural abscess
    - Correct coagulation abnormalities and consider surgical clot evacuation for epidural hematoma
    - Surgery may be indicated to treat the primary problem and to stabilize the spinal column

Prognosis/Complications

- Acute loss of spinal cord function, regardless of cause, has <10% chance of any recovery
- Paraparesis or quadraparesis existing for >24 hours has virtually no chance of recovery, regardless of treatment
- Progressive loss of neurologic function is usually stopped, but rarely reversed, with appropriate treatment
- Patients with significant loss of neurologic function are at risk for multiple medical complications, including pneumonia, deep venous thrombosis, pulmonary embolism, decubiti, and sepsis

135. Degenerative Spinal Disease

Etiology/Pathophysiology

- Progressive degenerative changes of the spine predispose to disc herniation and/or spondylosis (bone spurs)
- Often a result of normal aging; however, may also be initiated (in the case of herniations) or accelerated (in the case of spondylosis) by an acute injury
- Incidence of degenerative disease is greatest in the lumbar spine followed by the cervical spine, due to weight-bearing characteristics of these spinal segments
    - Disc herniation is more common in the lumbar spine
    - Spondylosis is more common in the cervical spine
- >80 million people per year seek treatment for back or neck pain
- The presence of "red flags" may signal serious underlying causes of back pain
    - Age >50 or <20
    - Fever
    - Increased pain at night or at rest
    - Known malignancy
    - Immunosuppression
    - History of trauma
    - Abnormal neurologic exam
    - Pulsatile abdominal mass
    - Anticoagulation

Differential Dx

- Peripheral neuropathy
- Neuritis/neuralgia
- Nerve compression secondary to malignancy, epidural abscess, or hematoma
- Other causes of radicular pain (e.g., carpal tunnel syndrome, rotator cuff pathology, hip disease)
- Trauma
- Referred pain secondary to abdominal aortic aneurysm, peptic ulcer disease, pancreatitis, renal colic, or ischemic pathology

Presentation/Signs & Symptoms

- Back or neck pain (depending on the involved spinal segment), with or without radicular extremity involvement
- Numbness/tingling
- Limited range of motion
- Nerve stretch tests may elicit pain in affected patients
    - Straight leg raise test (lumbar)
    - Spurling's sign (cervical)
- Loss or asymmetry of reflexes and/or muscle strength
- Dermatomal sensory loss
- Neurologic deficits are rare (e.g., bowel or bladder incontinence, focal muscle weakness)

Diagnostic Evaluation

- History and physical exam, including detailed neurologic examination
- MRI may delineate lesions; however, there is often a poor correlation between MRI results and clinical symptoms (i.e., many patients with normal MRI results have severe symptoms, whereas many asymptomatic patients have very abnormal MRI results)
- Myelogram with CT is indicated in patients who cannot undergo MRI (e.g., too large to fit into the MRI machine, claustrophobia) or if MRI results are equivocal
- Electromyography and nerve conduction velocity test

Treatment/Management

- Bed rest (however, >3 days of inactivity is *not* recommended)
- Limited activity for 2–3 weeks
- Analgesics and anti-inflammatory medications (e.g., acetaminophen, NSAIDs, COX-2 inhibitors)
- Muscle relaxants
- Steroids may be used in severe cases (administer for 6–7 days with tapering doses)
- Physical therapy, chiropractic manipulation, and adjunctive modalities (e.g., heat, ultrasound)
- Epidural steroid injections may be used in patients who have not responded to the above therapies and surgery is not an option
- Surgery may be indicated if the patient fails 4–6 weeks of conservative management or develops clear symptoms or signs of neurologic loss

Prognosis/Complications

- Most cases are self-limited with short-lived symptoms and require minimal treatment
- >80% of patients will recover within 4–6 weeks with conservative management alone
- <10% require surgery
- Long-term surgical success is approximately 70%
- Approximately 5% of patients who undergo surgery will develop chronic pain (post-laminectomy syndrome)
- Patients requiring surgical intervention have 2–3 times increased risk of recurrent or new problems

136. Spinal Stenosis

Etiology/Pathophysiology

- Most often due to degenerative changes with hypertrophy of the facet joints and supporting ligaments, resulting in gradual narrowing of the spinal canal with cord or nerve root impingement
- Most commonly seen after sixth decade of life
- Known as pseudoclaudication because symptoms imitate those of vascular claudication
  - Vascular claudication (i.e., peripheral vascular disease) generally presents with unilateral symptoms; spinal stenosis presents with bilateral symptoms

Differential Dx

- Cervical stenosis
  - Tumor
  - Motor neuron disease (e.g., amyotrophic lateral sclerosis)
- Lumbar stenosis
  - Vascular claudication
  - Disc disease
  - Synovial cyst
  - Tumor

Presentation/Signs & Symptoms

- Cervical stenosis
  - Neck pain and bilateral arm pain
  - Clumsiness of hands
  - Gait abnormalities
  - Lhermitte's phenomena: Paresthesias upon neck flexion
  - Intrinsic hand muscle atrophy in advanced cases
  - Myelopathy with pathologic reflexes
- Lumbar stenosis
  - Back pain, bilateral leg pain, and numbness
  - Exacerbated by exertion
  - Relieved by rest and lumbar flexion
  - Focal neurologic deficits
  - Bowel/bladder incontinence (rare)

Diagnostic Evaluation

- MRI will identify 90% of cases
- CT myelogram if unable to undergo MRI (e.g., too large to fit in MRI machine, claustrophobia)
- Electromyography and nerve conduction velocity studies
- Somatosensory evoked potentials
- Vascular Doppler studies may be indicated to differentiate spinal stenosis from vascular claudication

Treatment/Management

- NSAIDs and epidural steroid injections are the initial treatments; when started before surgery, these have been shown to improve outcomes
- Surgery (lumbar or cervical decompression) may be indicated if conservative medical management fails or if significant neurologic symptoms or signs are present

Prognosis/Complications

- >60% of cases will have symptomatic relief with conservative medical management
- Of those who undergo surgery, >80% will have adequate symptom relief
- Pre-existing neurologic deficits rarely improve with surgery; however, surgical correction will markedly lessen the chance of significant progression
- Potential complications of surgery include infection, CSF leakage, and new or worsened neurologic deficits (e.g., numbness, weakness, paralysis, pain, bowel/bladder dysfunction)

Orthopedic Surgery

Section 15

SCOTT KAHAN, MD
RICHARD F. FRISCH, MD

137. Orthopedic Anatomy, Facts, and Pearls

Anatomy of Long Bones
- Diaphysis (shaft): The long axis of a bone
- Metaphysis: End of the shaft of long bones, where it meets the epiphysis
- Physis: The growth plate
- Epiphysis: The ends of bone; articular cartilage covers the joint surface of each epiphysis

Secondary Nerve and Artery Injuries Frequently Associated with Orthopedic Injuries
- Shoulder dislocation may result in axillary nerve damage
- Humerus fracture may result in radial nerve or brachial artery damage
- Elbow dislocation may result in ulnar nerve, medial nerve, or brachial artery damage
- Hip dislocation may result in sciatic nerve damage or disruption of the arterial supply to the femoral head
- Posterior knee dislocation may result in peroneal nerve or popliteal artery damage

Orthopedic Emergencies
- Open fractures or dislocations
- Vascular or nerve injury
- Compartment syndromes
- Acute osteomyelitis or septic arthritis
- Hip dislocations (require immediate reduction to avoid avascular necrosis of the femoral head)
- Knee dislocations
- Exsanguinating pelvic fractures

Common Dermatomes, Myotomes, and Movements
- C5: Shoulder abduction
- C5/6: Elbow flexion
- C7: Elbow and finger extension
- C8: Finger flexion
- T1: Finger abduction
- T5: Nipple sensation
- T10: Umbilicus sensation
- L1: Inguinal ligament, hip flexion
- L2/3: Hip adduction
- L3/4: Knee extension
- L4: Knee jerk reflex, ankle dorsiflexion
- L5: Big toe extension
- L5/S1: Ankle eversion, hip extension
- S1: Ankle jerk reflex
- S1/2: Ankle plantarflexion
- S4/5: Perianal sensation

138. General Approach to Fractures

Etiology/Pathophysiology

- Fractures may be traumatic, stress-related (overuse injuries), or pathologic (secondary to bone weakness due to tumor or osteoporosis)
- History of osteoporosis, Paget's disease, chronic steroid use, or end-stage renal disease increases fracture risk
- The fracture diagnosis is often easily identified; however, it is important not to miss associated injuries—be sure to focus on the area of injury, one joint distal to the injury, and one joint proximal to the injury
- Open fractures occur with disruption of the overlying skin
  - Grade I: Wound <1 cm in length
  - Grade II: Wound >1 cm but <10 cm; clean and without devitalized tissue
  - Grade III: Wound >10 cm in length or one that is grossly contaminated; periosteal stripping of the bone, vascular or neurologic injury, and soft tissue loss may occur
- Dislocation: Complete loss of contact between two articular surfaces
  - The direction of dislocation or subluxation is determined by the displacement of the distal part (e.g., an anterior knee dislocation refers to forward dislocation of the tibia from the femur)
- Subluxation: Articular surfaces still in partial contact but no longer with normal congruous alignment
- Diastasis: Joint subluxation with widening of articulation

Differential Dx

- Avulsion fracture
- Impacted fracture
- Depressed fracture
- Pathologic fracture
- Stress fracture
- Ligamentous injury
- Tendon injury

Presentation/Signs & Symptoms

- Assess passive and active range of motion of the surrounding joints
- Circulatory status must be evaluated by palpating pulses, assessing capillary refill, and noting skin color
- Evaluate the neurologic system in terms of sensation, voluntary movement, and deep tendon reflexes
- Evaluate past medical history for pre-existing conditions that may alter management (e.g., diabetes mellitus)
- Broken skin lesions, lacerations, or superficial wounds may indicate an open fracture

Diagnostic Evaluation

- X-ray of the affected area requires at least two views at right angles to each other (e.g., A/P and lateral views) and views of one joint distal and one joint proximal to the area of injury to assess for associated injuries
  - Note length discrepancy (shortening of the bone)
  - Note angulation of the distal fracture piece
  - Note rotation of the bone due to the fracture
  - Note displacement of distal bone piece >50% from normal
  - Note soft tissue involvement (e.g., retained foreign bodies)
- Note fracture type
  - Transverse fracture: Perpendicular to the long axis of bone
  - Oblique fracture: Fracture line at oblique angle to the long axis of bone
  - Spiral fracture: Severe oblique fracture in which the fracture plane rotates along the long axis of bone; caused by a twisting injury
  - Segmental fracture: More than one fracture along the bone
  - Comminuted fracture: Fracture in more than two pieces

Treatment/Management

- General fracture management: Immobilize the affected area (including the joint above and below the injury), administer analgesia (NSAIDs and/or narcotics), ice, compression, and elevation
- Perform frequent neurovascular checks, particularly before and after any movement or reduction
- Infection prophylaxis as necessary
  - Tetanus prophylaxis
  - IV antibiotics directed against gram positives and anaerobes (e.g., first generation cephalosporin)
  - Open fractures require anti-staphylococcal coverage
- Wound lavage of open fractures within 6 hrs of injury
- Surgical debridement of devitalized or infected tissue
- Immobilization with a plaster splint and ace bandage (be aware that early circumferential casting may compromise blood supply)
- Dislocations, rotational deformities, and angulation deformities may require reduction under sedation

Prognosis/Complications

- Consult othopedics early
- Early complications include tendon injury, infection, compartment syndrome, hemorrhage, or neurovascular deficit
- Late complications include malunion, nonunion, delayed union, avascular necrosis, arthritis, neurovascular deficits, osteomyelitis, pulmonary embolus, and poor functional outcome

ORTHOPEDIC SURGERY

139. Pediatric Fractures

Etiology/Pathophysiology

- Fractures often occur at the physis (the weakest component of bone)
- Ligament injuries are uncommon in children (the physis is weaker than the ligaments; thus, fractures generally occur before the ligament tears)
- Salter-Harris classification of fractures that occur through the growth plate (physis) in children; physeal fractures may compromise normal growth
    - Type I: Fracture through the physis only (X-rays are often normal)
    - Type II (most common): Fracture through the physis and metaphysis
    - Type III: Fracture through the physis and epiphysis, and into the joint
    - Type IV: Fracture of the metaphysis, physis, and epiphysis
    - Type V: Crush injury of the physis (often misdiagnosed as type I)
- Complete (most common) fracture: Both sides of cortex are disrupted—may be spiral, transverse, oblique, or comminuted
- Buckle fracture: Incomplete disruption of the cortex, resulting in compression and bulging deformity of the cortex
- Greenstick fracture: Incomplete fracture with unilateral cortical fracture and bending of the opposite cortex
- Plastic deformity: Stress on the bone results in a bowing or bending deformity while the cortex remains intact
- Toddler's fracture: Oblique distal tibia fracture in infants

Differential Dx

- Radial head subluxation
- Transient hip tenosynovitis (hip pain following URI)
- Legg-Calvé-Perthes (avascular necrosis of femoral head)
- Osgood-Schlatter (apophysitis caused by repetitive traction to the tibial tuberosity)
- Slipped capital femoral epiphysis (groin or hip pain in an adolescent)

Presentation/Signs & Symptoms

- Pain, tenderness, and swelling
- Refusal to use the extremity or to bear weight
- Ecchymosis
- Tenderness over any physis (even with negative X-rays) is presumptively diagnosed as a Salter-Harris type I fracture
- Pediatric bones (more so than adult bones) are more likely to deform without breaking
- Radial head subluxation (Nursemaid's elbow) classically presents with the arm held in flexion and pronation

Diagnostic Evaluation

- Maintain a high index of suspicion for child abuse
- Plain X-rays will identify diaphyseal, metaphyseal, and Salter-Harris fractures (except type I and type V)
    - X-rays of Salter-Harris type I injuries are often initially normal; obtain follow-up X-rays 10–14 days after injury to attempt to identify these injuries
    - If fracture is at or near growth plate, X-rays should be done on both extremities to compare anatomy

Treatment/Management

- Analgesia with NSAIDs and narcotics
- Open fractures require tetanus immunization and anti-staphylococcal antibiotics
- Immediate reduction should be attempted for all displaced fractures
- Salter-Harris types I and II may be splinted to immobilize the joint above and below the fracture
- Salter-Harris types III, IV, and V fractures may require further treatment
- Displaced epiphyseal fractures, intra-articular fractures, open fractures, or fractures unable to be reduced appropriately will often require open reduction with internal fixation

Prognosis/Complications

- Complications include non-union, deformity, and growth arrest
- Salter-Harris fracture outcomes
    - I, II: Good healing, normal growth
    - III, IV: Increased risk of growth disruption
    - V: Growth complications are common
    - Increase in fracture severity results in increase in growth complications

140. Compartment Syndrome

Etiology/Pathophysiology

- A life-threatening condition caused by increased pressure in a closed anatomic space
- Compartments have a fixed volume; external constriction or introduction of excess fluid into the compartment increases pressure in the compartment
- Decreased perfusion occurs as the tissue compartmental pressure exceeds perfusion pressure, ultimately resulting in tissue hypoxia, anaerobic metabolism, and ischemic necrosis
- Causes include trauma (e.g., fracture, crush injury), vascular compromise, reperfusion injury, edema (e.g., burns, nephrotic syndrome, envenomation), coagulopathies, external compression (e.g., MAST, casts, prolonged compression from falls)
  - Common injuries leading to compartment syndrome include supracondylar elbow fracture in children and proximal or midshaft tibial fracture
- Most common in the calf and forearm

Differential Dx

- Arterial injury
- Peripheral nerve injury
- Rhabdomyolysis
- Cellulitis
- Deep venous thrombosis
- Thrombophlebitis
- Gas gangrene
- Necrotizing fasciitis

Presentation/Signs & Symptoms

- Pain
  - Diffuse, intense pain
  - Out of proportion to exam
  - May occur at rest
  - Exacerbated by movement (including passive movement), touch, elevation, or muscle stretch
- Paresthesias (due to nerve ischemia)
- Pallor
- Pressure (palpable tenseness in the affected compartment)
- Pulselessness may be a late finding— however, since compartment syndrome is a disorder of the microvasculature, the major vessels are not often affected
- Paralysis
- Poikilothermia (cool limb)

Diagnostic Evaluation

- History and clinical suspicion should prompt immediate diagnostic testing—physical exam is not reliable enough to rule out the diagnosis
- Intracompartment pressure measurement should be performed if the diagnosis is suspected
  - Pressure >20 mmHg is abnormal
  - Pressure >30 may indicate compartment syndrome
  - Pressure >40 is diagnostic for compartment syndrome
- Measure serum creatinine phosphokinase, myoglobin, and urine myoglobin to rule out rhabdomyolysis
- Coagulation studies (PT/PTT/INR) may be ordered to rule out underlying coagulopathies
- X-ray may show gas (due to infection) or other abnormalities in the affected extremity
- Ultrasound may be used to rule out DVT, but is not diagnostic for compartment syndrome

Treatment/Management

- Keep extremities level with the body (extremity elevation decreases limb mean arterial pressure without affecting intracompartmental pressure, thereby further decreasing perfusion)
- IV hydration and supplemental O$_2$ administration
- Maintain adequate urine volume and consider urine alkalinization to ensure removal of myoglobin
- Serial exams and pressure measurements
- Fasciotomy is the definitive therapy
  - Indicated for intracompartmental pressure >45 mmHg or within 10–30 mmHg of diastolic blood pressure
  - Should be done within 4 hours of injury to prevent permanent tissue injury
- Amputation is indicated to prevent gangrene if fasciotomy cannot be performed prior to muscle death

Prognosis/Complications

- Complications associated with untreated compartment syndrome include muscle necrosis and permanent nerve damage to the affected area
  - Irreversible tissue death can occur within 4–12 hours, depending on the tissue type and compartment pressures
  - Ischemic muscle contractures may develop after prolonged ischemia
  - Myoglobinuria occurs after reperfusion of the damaged tissue following fasciotomy
  - Death may occur secondary to infections or cardiac arrhythmias (due to hyperkalemia from tissue death)

141. Osteomyelitis

Etiology/Pathophysiology

- Infection of the bone
- Occurs due to hematogenous spread in 90% of cases; other etiologies include direct inoculation (e.g., trauma, surgery) and direct spread from a local soft tissue infection (e.g., diabetic foot ulcer)
    - *Staphylococcus aureus* causes >50% of cases
    - Gram-negative rods (e.g., *Pseudomonas, Salmonella, Serratia, E. coli*)
    - Anaerobes (especially in diabetics)
    - *Staphylococcus epidermidis* (especially in prosthetic joints)
    - Fungi (especially in immunocompromised patients)
    - *M. tuberculosis* (Pott's disease of the spine)
    - *Pasteurella* (cat or dog bites)
- High risk patients include those with diabetes, peripheral vascular disease, and IV drug use
- In adults, osteomyelitis most commonly occurs in the vertebrae
- In children, osteomyelitis usually occurs in the metaphyses of long bones
- Important cause of fever of unknown origin

Differential Dx

- Cellulitis
- Bone infarction
- Soft tissue infection (e.g., abscess)
- Trauma
- Fracture
- Gout
- Septic arthritis
- Degenerative joint disease
- Rheumatoid arthritis
- Metastatic cancer
- Bone tumor (e.g., Ewing's sarcoma)

Presentation/Signs & Symptoms

- Localized bone pain (not relieved by rest) and tenderness
- Warmth, redness
- Swelling; no decline in swelling with elevation of limb for 2 hours
- Non-healing ulcer may be present—any ulcer more than 2 weeks old should raise suspicion of osteomyelitis
- Systemic symptoms may be present (e.g., fever, chills, malaise, anorexia, nausea, vomiting)
- Children more commonly present with acute systemic infection; often they will refuse to use the limb or have decreased weight bearing
- Infants may present with irritability and a red, warm, tender extremity

Diagnostic Evaluation

- Plain X-rays are often the first test ordered; however, they are rarely positive early (may require 10–21 days before bony changes are seen); may see periosteal elevation, lytic lesions, cortical changes, or frank bone destruction
- ESR elevation is highly sensitive for osteomyelitis; leukocytosis is less sensitive (neither are specific)
- Blood cultures are positive only in 50–60% of cases
- Needle aspiration or open bone biopsy with culture are the best means to identify causative organism(s)
    - Wound cultures are usually *not* helpful because they are often contaminated with multiple pathogens
- Bone scan is very sensitive but not specific (i.e., does not differentiate infection from tumor or fracture)
- CT scan is used to determine the extent of disease; however, it also is often negative early in the illness
- MRI is especially useful to evaluate osteomyelitis of the spine or epidural abscess

Treatment/Management

- Administer IV antibiotics for 4–6 weeks, followed by oral antibiotics
    - Begin empiric coverage with two drugs until results of cultures and gram stain are available
    - Always include anti-staphylococcal coverage (e.g., cefazolin, nafcillin, clindamycin, vancomycin)
    - Also cover gram negatives (e.g., third or fourth generation cephalosporin, gentamicin, ciprofloxacin, imipenem)
    - Consider adding anaerobic coverage in diabetic patients (e.g., penicillin/anti-penicillinase, clindamycin)
    - Tailor antibiotics once Gram stain, cultures, and sensitivities are available
- Surgical drainage/debridement is indicated emergently in open fractures and if symptoms do not improve within the first 48 hours (more likely to be required in diabetic foot infections)

Prognosis/Complications

- Good prognosis if detected early
- Rule out septic joint involvement in all cases, as this requires urgent debridement
- If antibiotics are not effective, check for sensitivity or uncommon pathogens
- If patient is unresponsive to therapy, amputation may be necessary
- Complications include pathologic fracture, vertebral collapse with spinal cord compression, bacteremia, and sepsis
- Osteomyelitis often must be diagnosed clinically, even if available imaging appears negative; if patients have a consistent history and physical, immediately draw cultures and begin antibiotics
- Educate patients to prevent further episodes, especially in diabetics with recurrent foot lesions

142. Septic Arthritis

Etiology/Pathophysiology

- Acute infection of the synovial space
- The most commonly involved joints are the knee, hip, and shoulder
- Hematogenous spread is most common
- Disseminated gonococcal infection is the most common cause of acute arthritis in adults younger than age 45
- Non-gonococcal bacterial arthritis is the most destructive type of acute monoarthritis
    - Risk factors include diabetes, immunosuppression, rheumatoid arthritis, IV drug use, and prostheses
    - *Staphylococcus aureus* is the most common organism (group B *streptococcus* is the most common cause in infants)
    - Other common organisms include gram-negative rods (especially pseudomonas and *E. coli*), *Streptococcus pneumoniae, Streptococcus pyogenes, Borrelia, Mycobacterium tuberculosis,* and *Pasteurella* (dog/cat bites)
    - Fungi and viruses may produce a more chronic, subacute presentation
- Women are at higher risk during menses

Differential Dx

- Fracture
- Hemarthrosis
- Foreign body
- Rheumatoid arthritis
- Osteoarthritis
- Avascular necrosis
- Disseminated tuberculosis
- Reactive arthritis
- Reiter's syndrome
- Gout
- Pseudogout
- Lyme disease
- Diagnoses specific to the involved joint (e.g., meniscal rupture)

Presentation/Signs & Symptoms

- Mono- or oligoarticular arthritis
- Warmth, redness, and tenderness around the affected joint
- Decreased range of motion
- Signs of synovitis (e.g., severe pain upon passive or active movement)
- Systemic symptoms may be present (e.g., fever, chills, malaise)
- Disseminated gonorrhea may present with migratory arthritis, vesiculopustular lesions on fingers, tenosynovitis, and urethral discharge

Diagnostic Evaluation

- Laboratory studies are rarely useful (WBC and ESR may be elevated by any cause of inflammation) and may be normal
- Joint aspiration and analysis is performed in most patients
    - WBC >50,000 suggests an infectious etiology
    - WBC <50,000 suggests an inflammatory or autoimmune etiology (e.g., osteoarthritis, rheumatoid arthritis)
    - WBC <2000 suggests a non-inflammatory etiology
    - Gram stain and culture is positive in only 75% of cases
    - Presence of crystals suggests gout (needle-shaped, negatively birefringent urate crystals) or pseudogout (rod-shaped, positively birefringent calcium pyrophosphate crystals)
- Cervical/urethral cultures if gonorrhea is suspected
- Consider testing for syphilis, Lyme disease, and HIV
- X-rays may show fracture, tumor, effusion, or signs of osteomyelitis, osteoarthritis, or gout

Treatment/Management

- Begin empiric IV antibiotic coverage to cover *Staphylococcus aureus* and *Neisseria gonorrhea*
    - Nafcillin plus third generation cephalosporin (e.g., ceftriaxone, cefotaxime) or ciprofloxacin are good choices
    - Prosthetic joint involvement requires vancomycin plus gram-negative coverage (e.g., ciprofloxacin, gentamicin, cefipime)
    - Tailor antibiotics based on Gram stain and/or culture
- Treatment usually lasts 14 days (3–4 weeks for pyogenic organisms)
- Arthrotomy and open drainage may be necessary (especially for septic shoulder and hip)

Prognosis/Complications

- Failure to recognize a septic joint will lead to joint destruction and possible systemic sepsis and death
- Excellent prognosis when antibiotics are started early
- If *N. gonorrhea* is the causative organism, treat for chlamydia as well and screen for other STDs

143. Tumors of Bone

Etiology/Pathophysiology

- Primary benign tumors are more common than malignant tumors
  - Bony tumors include osteoid osteoma and osteoblastoma
  - Cartilaginous tumors include osteochondroma, chondroblastoma, and enchondroma
  - Other benign tumors include fibromas, fibrous dysplasia, bone cysts, and giant cell tumors
- Primary malignant tumors are rare
  - Osteosarcoma is the most common primary malignant bone tumor
  - Malignant tumors of bone marrow origin include Ewing's sarcoma, multiple myeloma, plasmacytoma, and leukemia
- Metastases are much more common than primary tumors
  - Often secondary to cancers of the prostate, breast, lungs, thyroid, and kidney

Differential Dx

- Osteomyelitis
- Traumatic bone injury
- Stress fracture
- Myositis ossificans
- Arthritis

Presentation/Signs & Symptoms

- Pain is the most common complaint
  - Deep, aching pain
  - Not relieved by rest
  - Night pain is often present
- Swelling
- Decreased range of motion
- Palpable mass may be present
- Large tumors may cause radicular symptoms as they impede on nerves
- Malignancies may present with constitutional symptoms (e.g., fever, chills, weight loss)
- Malignant tumors are more likely to be symptomatic; however, some benign tumors (e.g., osteoid osteoma) and large tumors are often symptomatic
- Pathologic fractures may occur

Diagnostic Evaluation

- X-rays identify the location and characteristics of the tumor
  - General findings include bone expansion, calcification, lytic change, and periosteal reaction
  - Signs consistent with benign lesions include well-circumscribed sclerotic borders
  - Signs consistent with malignant lesions include moth-eaten appearance, cortical disruption, expansion within the bone, or extension to surrounding soft tissue
- CT and/or MRI are used for staging and to better delineate areas in question
  - CT is best for benign bony lesions
  - MRI will better characterize malignant lesions
- Bone biopsy is indicated for any lesion that is not assured to be benign based on radiographic and clinical findings
- Metastatic workup should include CBC with differential, ESR, CRP, chemistries, calcium, phosphate, LFTs, TFTs, PSA, SPEP/UPEP, chest X-ray, chest CT, bone scan

Treatment/Management

- Observation may be appropriate for asymptomatic benign tumors
- Benign tumors that are enlarging or cause unbearable pain should undergo full metastatic workup and possible resection
- All malignant tumors are generally excised and may require chemotherapy and/or radiation

Prognosis/Complications

- Osteosarcoma, though rare, tend to metastasize widely; approximately 20% of patients have pulmonary metastases at the time of diagnosis; long-term survival is 60%
- Patients with suspected malignant tumors should be referred for biopsy to an orthopedic oncologist in the facility where definitive management is to occur

Pediatric Surgery

MICHAEL G. SCHEIDLER, MD

144. Omphalocele

Etiology/Pathophysiology

- Abdominal wall defects comprise a spectrum of defects that extend from the sternum (ectopia cordis) to the pubis (exstrophy of the bladder) of which gastroschisis and omphaloceles are the most common
- Characterized by a defect of the umbilical ring and medial segments of the lateral abdominal wall folds, resulting in herniation of abdominal viscera through the umbilicus
  - In contrast to gastroschisis, the herniated viscera is contained within the peritoneal sac
  - Herniated organs may include the liver, intestines, and bladder
- Associated anomalies are common (up to 40–80% of patients)
  - Cardiac anomalies (e.g., tetralogy of Fallot, atrial septal defect) occur in up to 25% of patients
  - Other associated anomalies include Pentalogy of Cantrell, cloacal exstrophy, Beckwith-Wiedemann syndrome, various trisomy syndromes, and genitourinary anomalies
- No definitive etiologic factors have been identified although many have been hypothesized (e.g., smoking, young mothers)
- Intestines are always malrotated

Differential Dx

- Gastroschisis
- Umbilical hernia

Presentation/Signs & Symptoms

- Obvious herniation of abdominal contents at the umbilicus
- Because a membranous sac is present, the bowel is well protected; these children do not have the initial evaporative fluid losses associated with gastroschisis
- The sac may be ruptured in up to 10% of cases

Diagnostic Evaluation

- Prenatal diagnosis is frequently possible
  - Elevated maternal serum α-fetoprotein
  - Prenatal ultrasound
- Differentiate from gastroschisis
  - Defect through the umbilicus rather than the abdominal wall
  - Larger defect than gastroschisis
  - Cord inserts into sac
  - Defect contains bowel and liver
- Due to the increased risk of anomalies, cardiac echocardiography and renal ultrasound are indicated

Treatment/Management

- Emergent management of hypothermia
- Maintenance IV fluid replacement need not be as great as in gastroschisis since the peritoneal sac envelopes the viscera
- Prophylactic antibiotics
- In cases of respiratory distress, obtain an airway, place orogastric tube to decompress the bowel, provide sedation, and begin mechanical ventilation
- Surgical repair is not emergent unless congenital malrotation with a midgut volvulus is present with signs of intestinal obstruction
- Small omphaloceles (<6 cm) can be repaired in a single-staged procedure; larger defects require gradual reduction into the abdominal cavity
- Conservative management with topical silver sulfadiazine may be attempted for infants with an intact membrane who have severe cardiac or respiratory defects

Prognosis/Complications

- Postoperative ileus persists for up to 1 month and nutritional support is required
- Overall mortality is higher in omphalocele (15–20%) compared to gastroschisis
- Associated congenital anomalies are the major cause of death (30–40% mortality)
- Complications may occur early (e.g., catheter sepsis, gastroesophageal reflux, short gut syndrome) or late (e.g., post-surgical obstruction, growth delay)
- Infectious complications are increased if sac is ruptured at presentation
- Congenital malrotation with midgut volvulus accompanied by signs of intestinal obstruction is often seen in children with omphalocele and is a surgical emergency

145. Gastroschisis

Etiology/Pathophysiology

- Abdominal wall defects comprise a spectrum of defects that extend from the sternum (ectopia cordis) to the pubis (exstropy of the bladder) of which gastroschisis and omphaloceles are the most common
- Characterized by a defect in the abdominal wall lateral to the umbilical cord and involving the lateral aspect of the umbilical ring, resulting in herniation of the intestinal contents through the abdominal wall
    - In contrast to omphalocele, the herniated viscera is not protected by the peritoneal sac
    - Herniated organs may include the stomach and small bowel
- Associated anomalies are rare (intestinal atresia occurs in 10–15% of cases)
- No definitive etiologic factors have been identified although many have been hypothesized (e.g., smoking, young mothers)
- Occurs between 10 and 12 weeks of gestation
- Normally, the midgut develops outside the abdominal cavity and rotates upon re-entering; in children with abdominal wall defects, the midgut does not re-enter and the intestines are always malrotated

Differential Dx

- Omphalocele
- Umbilical hernia

Presentation/Signs & Symptoms

- Obvious herniation of abdominal contents at birth
- Infants are often dehydrated and hypothermic due to insensible losses via the exposed gut

Diagnostic Evaluation

- Prenatal diagnosis is possible
    - Elevated maternal serum α-fetoprotein
    - Prenatal ultrasound
- Differentiate from omphalocele
    - Location of defect (to the right side of the umbilicus with the umbilical cord found on the left side of the sac)
    - Absence of peritoneal sac
    - Normal insertion of cord
    - Smaller defect than omphalocele
    - Frequently contains bowel (but never liver)

Treatment/Management

- Upon delivery and normal newborn resuscitation, place the lower half of the infant along with the viscera into a sterile bowel bag to prevent increased insensible fluid loss
- Obtain an airway in cases of respiratory distress, place orogastric tube to decompress bowel, and begin IV fluid administration, sedation, and mechanical ventilation
- Parenteral antibiotics to decrease the risk of sepsis
- Manage hypovolemia and hypothermia
- Immediate surgical correction is required
    - Defect can be closed primarily or by staged reduction
    - If closure creates undue tension or increased intra-abdominal pressure, a staged repair is required
    - Staged repair occurs by gradual reduction of the intestinal contents over 3–5 days; the fascial defect is then closed with or without a patch

Prognosis/Complications

- Postoperative ileus persists for up to 1 month and nutritional support is required
- Overall mortality of 10%
- Complications may occur early (e.g., catheter sepsis, gastroesophageal reflux, short gut syndrome) or late (e.g., post-surgical obstruction)
- Parenteral nutrition is required for several months
- Delayed onset of necrotizing enterocolitis is not uncommon and should be suspected if bloody stools are observed

146. Intestinal Atresia

Etiology/Pathophysiology

- Small intestine atresia may occur in the duodenum, jejunum, or ileum, resulting in intestinal obstruction
- Duodenal atresia is often associated with genetic conditions such as Down's syndrome
  - Thought to occur by failure of recanalization of the duodenal lumen
  - High incidence of associated anomalies (30% of affected patients have trisomy 21, 20% have congenital heart disease)
  - Majority of cases are limited to the first or second portion of the duodenum
  - 85% of cases are distal to the bile duct; thus, most affected infants have bilious emesis
- Jejunal and ileal atresia arise from in utero vascular accidents, intrauterine intussusception, or volvulus of ileum and are not associated with other major congenital anomalies

Differential Dx

- Ileus secondary to neonatal sepsis
- Malrotation with or without midgut volvulus
- Meconium ileus/plug
- Colonic atresia
- Total colonic aganglionosis (Hirschsprung's disease)

Presentation/Signs & Symptoms

- Bilious vomiting is present in most cases
- Feeding intolerance
- Frequent episodes of apnea and bradycardia
- Abdominal distention is most prominent with distal atresia

Diagnostic Evaluation

- Polyhydramnios on prenatal ultrasound is a marker of intestinal obstruction
- Abdominal X-ray showing a "double-bubble" sign is diagnostic of duodenal obstruction (distended stomach and duodenum with no gas in the rest of the abdomen)
  - If distal gas is present, differentiate a partial duodenal obstruction (e.g., duodenal web or stenosis) from a midgut volvulus (which is a surgical emergency)
- In cases of jejunoileal atresia, a contrast enema is helpful to determine the site of obstruction (large versus small bowel) and to locate the position of the cecum to rule out malrotation
- Upper GI studies are routinely obtained for duodenal atresia
- A thorough evaluation for associated abnormalities (e.g., congenital heart defects) is necessary in cases of duodenal atresia

Treatment/Management

- Duodenal atresia is corrected surgically via a duodenoduodenostomy
  - Care is taken to avoid the ampulla of Vater
  - The continuity of the remaining intestines is tested by injecting saline into the bowel until it reaches the colon
- Jejunoileal atresia is corrected by primary anastomosis of the two blind ends
  - The distal end is generally small; thus, an oblique transection is performed to increase the anastomotic size
  - If the size discrepancy is still too large, the proximal bowel can be tapered along the antimesenteric border to decrease the size of the lumen

Prognosis/Complications

- Survival rates exceed 85–90% for all intestinal atresia
- Anastomotic leaks occur in <5% of cases
- The most common complication is pneumonia and catheter sepsis

147. Pyloric Stenosis

Etiology/Pathophysiology

- Hypertrophy of the pylorus, resulting in a functional gastric outlet obstruction
- Incidence is estimated at 1% of infants with a male predominance (4:1)
- White > African-American > Asian
- Etiology is unknown; may be related to an abnormal enteric nervous system, decreased neuropeptides, decreased ganglion cells, or decreased nitric oxide synthase

Differential Dx

- Overfeeding or formula intolerance
- Gastroesophageal reflux
- Pylorospasm
- Metabolic disorders
- Malrotation

Presentation/Signs & Symptoms

- Presents at 3–6 weeks of age
- Progressively increasing projectile, non-bilious emesis
- Dehydration
- Olive-shaped abdominal mass is palpable in >80% of cases
    - Best palpated with infant supine while nursing a bottle

Diagnostic Evaluation

- Physical exam is diagnostic in most cases
- Ultrasound is the diagnostic modality of choice if uncertainty exists following clinical exam
    - Criteria for pyloric stenosis includes pyloric muscle thickness >3 mm or pyloric canal length >17 mm
- Upper GI series may show a "string sign," revealing the narrowed pyloric channel
- Gastric loss of Cl⁻ and H⁺ results in a hypokalemic, hypochloremic, metabolic alkalosis
- Due to the severe dehydration and hypovolemia, patients have acidic urine despite serum alkalosis (paradoxic aciduria)

Treatment/Management

- Adequate rehydration with appropriate potassium supplementation
- Pyloromyotomy (Ramstedt operation) is the definitive treatment
    - Right upper quadrant incision, umbilical incision, or laparoscopy may be used

Prognosis/Complications

- Overall outcome is excellent; most children are discharged within 24 hours after surgery
- Duodenal perforation occurs in <1% of cases
    - Easy to repair if identified at the time of the initial procedure; however, morbidity increases substantially if perforation is not recognized
- Gastritis affects most infants to some degree but generally resolves without intervention

148. Intussusception

Etiology/Pathophysiology

- Telescoping of a proximal segment of intestine (intussusceptum) into the distal segment (intussuscipiens)
- 80% of cases are ileocecal intussusceptions
- 70% of cases occur in patients <1 year old (most common in infants 5–10 months)
- The most common abdominal emergency in infants
- There is a seasonal variation with the highest incidence in the spring (associated with gastroenteritis) and winter (associated with respiratory infections)
- There is a specific lead point in 2–8% of the children, often a Meckel's diverticulum or lymphoid hyperplasia

Differential Dx

- Appendicitis
- Gastroenteritis
- Mesenteric adenitis
- Volvulus
- Incarcerated hernia

Presentation/Signs & Symptoms

- Typical presentation is a previously healthy infant with sudden onset of severe, intermittent abdominal pain
- Vomiting
- Blood and mucus per rectum ("currant jelly" stools)
- Fits of screaming and diaphoresis
- Lethargy
- A palpable, sausage-shaped mass may be detected in the right lower quadrant
- Other findings may include fever and tachycardia

Diagnostic Evaluation

- Air contrast enema is diagnostic; often, the enema will reduce the intussusception
- Ultrasound with pneumatic decompression is operator dependent and has not gained widespread application; however, this method does limit radiation exposure and may be therapeutic

Treatment/Management

- Surgical reduction is necessary if pneumatic reduction is unavailable or unsuccessful
- Through a right lower quadrant incision, the intussuscepted bowel is pushed (not pulled); adhesive bands at the base of the intussusception are lysed and an appendectomy is performed

Prognosis/Complications

- Overall prognosis is excellent
  - 75–95% success rate with pneumatic reduction
  - <1% perforation rate with pneumatic reduction
- 5–10% of children will have a recurrence
- 90% of recurrences occur within the initial 24 hours following treatment; thus, hospital admission and observation is required

149. Meckel's Diverticulum

Etiology/Pathophysiology

- A true diverticulum of the bowel, located on the antimesenteric border within 100 cm of the ileocecal valve
- Results from the failure of the vitelline duct to regress during the 5th–7th week of fetal life
- Overall incidence is 2% with male predominance
- Blood supply to the Meckel's diverticulum is from the paired vitelline arteries
- Attached to the abdominal wall in <20% of cases
- Heterotropic mucosa is found in 15% of incidental diverticula and 60% of symptomatic diverticula (gastric mucosa is most common followed by pancreatic tissue)
- Known as the "disease of 2's":
  - –2% of population
  - –2 inches in length
  - –occurs 2 feet from ileocecal valve
  - –2 times more common in males
  - –contains 2 types of ectopic GI tissue (gastric and pancreatic)
  - –2 major complications: Bleeding and inflammation

Differential Dx

- Appendicitis
- Gastroenteritis
- Mesenteric adenitis
- Intussusception
- Duodenal ulcer

Presentation/Signs & Symptoms

- Most cases will present by 2 years of age
- Lower GI bleeding occurs in 25–40% of cases
  - –Painless bleeding in a child <5 years old strongly suggests the diagnosis
  - –Bleeding is usually episodic
  - –Gastric mucosa is almost always present
- Intestinal obstruction occurs in 25–35% of cases
  - –Intussusception
  - –Volvulus
- Meckel's diverticulitis occurs in 15–25% of cases, which may mimic appendicitis

Diagnostic Evaluation

- In cases of lower GI bleeding, a Technetium nuclear scan (Meckel's scan) is used to detect ectopic gastric mucosa
- In cases of obstruction, an ultrasound may detect an intussusception with a Meckel's diverticulum as the lead point

Treatment/Management

- Most cases are corrected surgically by a wedge excision of the diverticulum
- Broad-based diverticula may require ileal resection

Prognosis/Complications

- Overall prognosis is excellent, with no long-term consequences
- Asymptomatic diverticula may be resected if length >2 cm or if heterotropic mucosa is present

150. Biliary Atresia

Etiology/Pathophysiology

- Progressive destruction of bile ducts secondary to an inflammatory process
- Proposed causes include failure of recanalization of the bile duct, embryogenic defects, vascular insufficiency, or viral infections
- Incidence ranges from 1/10,000 to 1/12,000 live births, without racial predilection
- 10% of affected infants have associated congenital heart disease
- Biliary atresia is the most frequent indication for liver transplant among infants and children

Differential Dx

- Neonatal hepatitis
- Interlobular biliary hypoplasia
- α-1 antitrypsin deficiency
- Choledochal cyst
- Inspissated bile syndrome
- Spontaneous perforation of bile duct

Presentation/Signs & Symptoms

- Jaundice beyond the first 2 weeks of life
- Acholic stools
- Dark urine
- Hepatomegaly
- Splenomegaly (late)
- May present with anemia, malnutrition, and fat-soluble vitamin (A, D, E, K) deficiency
- Affected children generally have normal growth and development

Diagnostic Evaluation

- Laboratory tests should include liver function tests, urobilinogen, and lipoprotein-X
  - Elevated conjugated bilirubin (>20%)
- Abdominal ultrasound is used to determine for the presence and size of the gallbladder
- Nuclear scanning (HIDA scan) will demonstrate lack of bile excretion into the small intestine
- Liver biopsy will reveal bile stasis, widening of portal tracts, giant cell transformation, and focal necrosis of liver cells; at the porta hepatis, duct-like structures are infiltrated with inflammatory cells
- Laparotomy with cholangiogram may be necessary for definitive diagnosis

Treatment/Management

- Early surgery (before 3 months of age) is required
- Hepatic portoenterostomy (Kasai's procedure): Roux-en-Y limb of the jejunum is anastomosed to the porta hepatitis to re-establish bile flow
- Liver transplant may be indicated for progressive hepatic decompensation, refractory growth failure, hepatic synthetic dysfunction, development of coagulopathies, or intractable portal hypertension with GI hemorrhage

Prognosis/Complications

- Survival depends on age at initial operation; prognosis is improved if performed before 2 months of age
  - Without surgery, most children will die before 2 years of age
  - One-third have rapid progression of the disease as a neonate
  - One-third of patients do well until the teenage years but then progress to liver failure, necessitating liver transplantation
  - One-third of patients maintain good function and never experience difficulties
- Cholangitis is the most common (40–90%) and most serious complication
- Portal hypertension occurs in half of cases
- Bile flow at the time of operation is an independent predictor of outcome

151. Congenital Diaphragmatic Hernia

Etiology/Pathophysiology

- Failure of the posterolateral portion of the diaphragm to develop, resulting in persistence of the pleuroperitoneal canal (foramen of Bochdalek), which allows the abdominal viscera to herniate into the chest cavity
- 85–90% of hernias occur on the left (left side closes later than right side) and malrotation of the intestines is always present
- As a result of the abdominal viscera developing in the chest, pulmonary hypoplasia ensues with a significant reduction in the number of bronchopulmonary segments and development of pulmonary hypertension
- Incidence is estimated to be 1/4000–5000 live births

Differential Dx

- Bronchogenic cyst
- Cystic adenomatoid malformation
- Congenital pneumonia
- Intralobar pulmonary sequestration

Presentation/Signs & Symptoms

- Severe respiratory distress and cyanosis within minutes of birth
- Absent breath sounds on the affected side
- Scaphoid abdomen

Diagnostic Evaluation

- Prenatal ultrasound detects >50% of cases
- Chest X-ray shows bowel gas pattern in chest with displacement of mediastinum
- Hypercarbia and/or hypoxia

Treatment/Management

- Place orogastric tube to decompress the stomach
- Mild mechanical ventilation ("gentilation") to prevent barotrauma
- Permissive hypercapnia and to correct acidosis
- Operative repair with reduction of the herniated viscera and correction of the diaphragmatic defect should occur after stabilization of the infant
  - Transabdominal approach is the most common
  - Reduction of herniated viscera
  - Attempt primary approximation of upper and lower lips of the defect; may require prosthetic patch
- Extracorporeal membrane oxygenation (ECMO) may be used as a salvage maneuver in those unable to be managed by conventional measures

Prognosis/Complications

- Survival rates range from 50–75%, regardless of the management scheme
- Severely affected infants may develop chronic pulmonary disease secondary to pulmonary hypoplasia
- Gastroesophageal reflux occurs in up to 70% of these children; however, surgical treatment is needed in only 15% of cases
- Intestinal obstruction occurs in 20% of cases secondary to adhesions or midgut volvulus
- Recurrent hernias occurs in 10% of cases and are more common in those requiring a patch closure
- Growth retardation and developmental delays are common

152. Tracheoesophageal Fistula

Etiology/Pathophysiology

- A spectrum of congenital esophageal atresias with or without a fistula to the trachea
  - Type A: Esophageal atresia without fistula (8%)
  - Type B: Esophageal atresia with a fistula between the proximal esophagus and the trachea (2%)
  - Type C: Esophageal atresia with a fistula between the distal esophagus and the trachea (85%)
  - Type D: Esophageal atresia with a fistula between the proximal and distal portions of the esophagus and the trachea (1%)
  - Type E (commonly referred to as "H-type"): Isolated fistula between the esophagus and trachea (4%)
- Risks factors include first pregnancy, diabetic mothers, increasing maternal age, and prolonged oral contraceptive use
- Often associated with cardiovascular anomalies (35%), genitourinary anomalies (20%), gastrointestinal anomalies (24%), neurologic anomalies (10%), skeletal anomalies (13%), and VACTERL (25%)
- Incidence of 2.4/10,000 live births

Differential Dx

- Duodenal atresia
- Esophageal stenosis
- Esophageal web
- Malrotation

Presentation/Signs & Symptoms

- Most cases become symptomatic within the first few hours of life
- Excess salivation
- Regurgitation, choking, or coughing upon first feeding
- Cyanosis with and without feeding
- Inability to pass orogastric tube into the stomach
- Type E often has a delayed presentation and may present with recurrent pneumonias due to repeated pulmonary aspiration

Diagnostic Evaluation

- Prenatal detection is possible in about half of cases, with small or absent stomach bubble and polyhydramnios
- Confirm the diagnosis by a lateral chest X-ray with a firm tube through the mouth into the esophageal pouch (dilated with air)

Treatment/Management

- Pre-operative preparation requires broad-spectrum antibiotics and placement of a suction catheter into the proximal pouch to minimize aspiration
- Avoid intubation, which may cause abdominal distension via ventilation through the fistula, thereby increasing the risk of gastric perforation and respiratory distress
- Surgical correction involves division of the fistula from the trachea with primary repair of the esophagus
  - If the distance between the ends of the esophagus is too far apart for anastomosis, surgery may be delayed to allow for further growth; esophageal replacement with small bowel or colon interposition may be necessary

Prognosis/Complications

- Prognosis depends on the presence of cardiac defects and birth weight
  - Cardiac anomalies portend a poor prognosis
  - Low weight neonates (<1.5 kg) with major cardiac anomalies have the poorest survival (<10%)
- Early complications of surgical repair include anastomotic leak, esophageal stricture, and recurrent fistula
- Late complications include gastroesophageal reflux, tracheomalacia, dysfunctional peristalsis, and pseudodiverticulum formation

153. Necrotizing Enterocolitis

Etiology/Pathophysiology

- Ischemia and necrosis of the intestinal mucosa, which can progress to full thickness necrosis of the bowel
- Primarily seen in premature neonates
- The most common surgical emergency in newborns
  - Affects 1–8% of babies in the neonatal intensive care unit
  - 25–35% of cases require surgery
- 50% of cases involve a single area (most commonly the distal ileum)
- 30% of cases have multiple skip lesions
- 20% of cases have pan-intestinal involvement
- Etiology is unknown but many risk factors have been identified, including prematurity, feeding (>90% of affected premature infants were fed), and use of vasoconstrictive drugs (e.g., theophylline, indomethacin)

Differential Dx

- Ileus associated with neonatal sepsis
- Hirschsprung's disease
- Meconium ileus/plug

Presentation/Signs & Symptoms

- Usually presents in the first week of life or 3–7 days after the onset of initial enteral feeds
- Abdominal distention is the most frequent early sign
- Rectal bleeding
- Increased gastric residuals
- Bilious vomiting
- Non-specific signs include respiratory distress, temperature instability, and apnea/bradycardic episodes
- Sepsis

Diagnostic Evaluation

- A clinical diagnosis that requires a high index of suspicion
- Abdominal X-rays are the mainstay of evaluation
  - Ileus pattern
  - Pneumatosis intestinalis (intramural gas caused by enteric flora producing hydrogen) is pathognomonic
  - Portal venous air is associated with pan-involvement
  - Free fluid
  - Pneumoperitoneum (best viewed with a left lateral decubitus film)
  - Persistent dilated loop of small intestine
- Laboratory studies may reveal leukocytosis, anemia and thrombocytopenia (due to gram-negative sepsis), and progressive metabolic acidosis

Treatment/Management

- Place orogastric tube
- Administer antibiotics to cover the intestinal flora
- Laparotomy or peritoneal drainage (in neonates <1000 grams) are indicated if pneumoperitoneum, fixed intestinal loop, portal venous gas, or paracentesis with positive gram stain are present
- Resection with preservation of as much bowel as possible
  - Isolated disease is most commonly treated with formation of an ostomy
  - Multiple segmental disease (<50% of intestine involved) is treated by a proximal jejunostomy with distal repair; "patch, drain, and wait" effort to preserve bowel length
  - Pan-involvement (>75% involved) requires a high jejunostomy

Prognosis/Complications

- Minor complications include wound infection, incisional hernia, catheter infection, and cholestasis
- Major complications include death (40%), stricture (13%), short gut syndrome (10%), enterocutaneous fistula (6%), and recurrent necrotizing enterocolitis (5%)
- Patients with pan-intestinal involvement have significant mortality; 100% mortality in neonates <1000 grams
  - Most surviving patients develop short gut syndrome

154. Cryptorchidism

Etiology/Pathophysiology

- Cryptorchidism describes failure of the testes to descend into the scrotum
- Occurs more commonly in premature infants than full-term infants (30% versus 3%)
- The testes develop within the abdomen and then descend during the third trimester through the inguinal canal and into the scrotum
  - This descent is dependent on testosterone, pituitary factors, gubernaculum, and mechanical factors
- Normal descent may continue up to 1 year after birth; after 1 year, it is unlikely for the testes to descend
- There is a 7-fold increase in the risk of testicular malignancy in patients with cryptorchidism

Differential Dx

- Testicular agenesis
- Intrauterine testicular torsion

Presentation/Signs & Symptoms

- Absence of testicles in the scrotum
- The testicles may be palpated in the inguinal canal

Diagnostic Evaluation

- Determine if testicles are present in the abdomen via serologic measurements of hormone levels
- If a testis is not palpable in the scrotum or the inguinal canal, an ultrasound may be indicated to evaluate for the presence of an ipsilateral kidney; if the kidney is absent, the diagnosis is testicular agenesis rather than cryptorchidism
- Imaging to locate intra-abdominal testis is rarely indicated
- Diagnostic laparoscopy is useful in cases of non-palpable undescended testes to locate the abdominal testicular tissue

Treatment/Management

- If the testicles can be re-positioned into the scrotum, no further intervention is necessary
- Hormonal therapy with low dose hCG is controversial
- Testicles should be surgically placed into the scrotum at about 1 year of age, as further descent will not occur beyond 1 year
  - Palpable undescended testicles are treated by orchidopexy with creation of a subdartos pouch (95% success rate)
  - Non-palpable undescended testicles require diagnostic laparoscopy to locate the abdominal testicular tissue, followed by mobilization of the testicular tissue and placement into the scrotum (success rate >80%)

Prognosis/Complications

- The increased risk of testicular malignancy is not decreased by orchidopexy, but surveillance is made easier
- Higher incidence of infertility in these patients

Appendices

Appendix A

Advanced Trauma Life Support (ATLS®)
- The Advanced Trauma Life Support (ATLS®) Program is a licensed course of the American College of Surgeons designed to provide a reliable and safe method for emergent resuscitation and acute management of trauma and shock patients
- Trauma is the leading cause of death in the first 4 decades of life
    - There are 60 million traumatic injuries annually in the U.S.
    - 3.6 million trauma patients annually require hospitalization
    - 8.7 million trauma patients have temporary disability
    - 300,000 patients have permanent disability
- The hallmark of trauma management is a systematic team approach between physicians, nurses, medics, X-ray technicians, and respiratory therapists
- Assessment and management follows a prioritized, sequential four-phase management protocol according to the ATLS program

- ## Phase I: *Primary Survey* (the "ABCDE" of trauma care)
- Airway maintenance with proper cervical spine protection
- Breathing (adequacy of ventilation)
- Circulation with control of external hemorrhage
- Disability (rapid neurologic evaluation of level of consciousness and pupillary response)
- Exposure and environmental control (fully undress the patient and protect from hypothermia with warm blankets)

- ## Phase II: *Resuscitation*
- Secure and protect the airway
- Oxygenate and ventilate the patient, intubate if necessary
- Shock management (IV fluids, blood replacement, control of external bleeding)
- Manage life-threatening conditions identified in the primary survey
- Monitor the patient (ECG, pulse oximetry, blood pressure, blood gases, end-tidal CO_2 capnometry)
- Gastric and urinary catheters
- Diagnostic tests as necessary (chest and pelvic X-rays, abdominal ultrasound)

- ## Phase III: *Secondary Survey*
- Complete head-to-toe exam of the patient, including all anatomic regions of the body, rectal exam, pelvic exam in women, and "logrolling" the patient to examine the back
- Complete neurologic exam
- Reassess vital signs and evaluate the results of resuscitation

- ## Phase IV: *Definitive care and disposition*
- CT scans of head and/or abdomen if indicated
- Surgical repair of injuries and/or fractures
- Admit to intensive care unit if appropriate
- Transfer to trauma or specialized care center if appropriate

Appendix B

Principles of Mechanical Ventilation

Mechanical ventilation has developed as a critical intervention since its beginnings in the middle of the 20th century. Whether providing respiratory support for patients recovering from elective surgery or as a life saving procedure following cardiac arrest or multiple trauma, the role of properly applied mechanical ventilation cannot be overstated.

The role of the respiratory system is to facilitate the exchange of oxygen and carbon dioxide to meet metabolic demand. This function is performed through an intimate synergy between the cardiovascular and respiratory systems. Dysfunction at any level of the cardiopulmonary (alveolar-capillary) interface results in *respiratory distress*, and tachypnea is the first indication of dysfunction.

> Patients with severe disease may progress from tachypnea to a normal respiratory rate to apnea. Thus, using tachypnea as an indicator of respiratory performance can be misleading in patients who are developing severe respiratory distress. The differentiating clinical sign is their mental status: If tachypnea seems to be resolving, but without a concomitant improvement in mental status, the patient may actually be worsening. True improvement in respiratory status should be accompanied by lowered respiratory rate *and* normalizing mental status.

Respiratory failure ensues when compensatory mechanisms become inadequate to overcome the physiologic insults that disrupt gas exchange. Signs of respiratory failure include severe tachypnea, hyperpnea (to increase tidal volume), hypoxemia (as demonstrated by PaO_2 on ABG or SpO_2 on pulse oximetry), diaphoresis, and altered mental status.

Respiratory arrest occurs when compensatory mechanisms have failed and signs of respiratory failure are accompanied by an irregular respiratory pattern (apnea, hypopnea) and/or reduced mental status.

Indications for Mechanical Ventilation

Impaired ventilation (hypercarbic respiratory failure) and/or impaired oxygenation (hypoxic respiratory failure)

Impaired ventilation results from conditions that impair minute ventilation (respiratory rate x tidal volume), including dysfunction of chest wall compliance, respiratory muscle performance, or neurologic drive. Specific indications for mechanical ventilation include an increase in arterial carbon dioxide (pCO_2 >50), decreased mental status or Glasgow coma scale <8, acidosis, chest wall trauma (e.g., flail chest), and apnea. Additionally, increased upper airway resistance (e.g., large tongue, loss of 'strap muscle' tone, foreign body) or increased lower airway resistance (e.g., bronchitis, reactive airways disease, aspiration) contribute to impaired minute ventilation.

Impaired oxygenation results from mechanisms that disrupt the cardiopulmonary interface, including pulmonary edema, ARDS, inhalation injury, aspiration, and severe tachypnea. These conditions result in increased intrapulmonary shunting and ventilation/perfusion mismatching. The delivery of high flow O_2 without an increase in oxygen saturation (pulse oximetry) should alert the clinician that significant intrapulmonary shunting is occurring. Also note that severe hypoxemia may occur in the absence of pulmonary disease, due to anemia (anemic hypoxia) or cardiac failure (ischemic hypoxia).

Mechanical Ventilators

The rapid development of ventilator hardware and software in the past 20 years coupled with our understanding of the pathophysiology of lung injury has dramatically improved care of mechanically ventilated patients. Current ventilators include complex servo-sensor mechanisms (patient-ventilator feedback) to optimize patient comfort and patient-ventilator interaction. Current ventilators allow nearly every facet of the respiratory cycle (inspiration-exhalation) to be prescribed.

Appendix B

Modes of Ventilation

The initiation and termination signal of each breath is the foundation of every mode of ventilation (how breathing is cycled). Modes of ventilation may be volume-cycled, time-cycled, or pressure-limited.

In volume-cycled modes, the tidal volume and respiratory rate are manipulated, leaving peak inspiratory pressure (PIP) as the necessary indicator of lung and chest wall compliance. Thus, PIP must be monitored as an index of patient status in volume-cycled modes.

In time-cycled and pressure-limited modes, the PIP and inspiratory times are prescribed, leaving tidal volume as the necessary indicator of lung and chest wall compliance. Thus, tidal volume must be monitored as an index of patient status in time-cycled and pressure-limited modes.

Types of Ventilation

Types of ventilation include assist control ventilation (ACV), controlled mandatory ventilation (CMV), pressure support ventilation (PSV), synchronized intermittent mandatory ventilation (SIMV), and pressure-controlled ventilation (PCV).

Assist control is a volume-cycled mode and is the preferred method of mechanical ventilation, as it requires a lower work of breathing. In this mode, breaths initiated by the patient are supported by positive pressure breaths at a prescribed tidal volume. ACV requires real-time, hands-on patient assessment. A backup rate of 10 breaths per minute is usually set in case the patient does not initiate a breath (e.g., due to oversedation or pharmacologic paralysis), essentially resulting in controlled mechanical ventilation (as below). It should be used with caution in agitated and tachypneic patients as barotrauma and respiratory alkalosis may ensue.

CMV eliminates patient involvement in breathing by design (the ventilator does all the work of breathing). Respiratory rate and either tidal volume or PIP are prescribed. Clinically, ACV in a deeply sedated or paralyzed patient becomes CMV.

In PSV, the breaths are initiated by the patient and the ventilator is set to deliver a prescribed PIP. The rate is patient-determined. Tidal volume is a function of lung and chest wall compliance and must be monitored as an index of patient status. PSV may be combined on contemporary ventilators with other modes. A rescue rate must be prescribed to compensate for apnea.

In SIMV, volume (in volume-cycled modes) or PIP (in time-cycled and pressure-limited modes) is prescribed. Through computerized servo mechanisms, patients can breathe between prescribed breaths and report great comfort. SIMV can be combined with other modes, such as PSV. SIMV does require more work than ACV.

PCV is historically the mode of choice for neonatal mechanical ventilation, as the highly compliant chest wall of neonates is often ineffective at maintaining the balance between elastic recoil and atelectasis. PCV, by combining a limited PIP with control of inspiratory time, optimizes mean airway pressure and oxygenation while minimizing volutrauma and barotrauma. PIP and inspiratory time are prescribed. Exhaled tidal volume is a function of lung and chest wall compliance and must be monitored as an index of patient status. As most intensivists favor using volume-cycled ventilation initially, the rapidity with which a patient requires pressure-limited mode of mechanical ventilation is a relative index of lung disease severity.

Continuous Positive Airway Pressure (CPAP) is an adjunct for intubated patients who are breathing on their own. With CPAP, patient breaths are supported by a prescribed constant end-expiratory pressure and can be combined with PSV.

Initiation and Maintenance of Mechanical Ventilation

Mechanical ventilation should be initiated with the goals of optimum gas exchange, patient-ventilator synchrony, improved cardiac performance, and patient comfort. Physiologically, the natural propensity of the chest wall is to "expand," whereas the natural tendency of the lungs is atelectasis. Where these forces of elastic recoil and atelectasis are in equilibrium is known as the functional residual capacity (FRC). The FRC facilitates tidal breathing and allows flexibility in the event that minute ventilation needs to be augmented with more than tidal breathing. The volume below which atelectasis is favored is the closing volume. At tidal breathing, FRC is always greater than closing volume. Tracheal intubation and positive pressure breathing eliminates the balance between elastic recoil and atelectasis and lowers FRC, favoring atelectasis.

Controversy has raged for decades over the optimum mode and style of mechanical ventilation to minimize iatrogenic lung injury. Elements of disagreement surrounded whether excessive pressure or tidal volumes were the culprit. It now appears that these components of mechanical ventilation are inextricably linked and probably both play a role. Recent data has added a new word to the language of acute lung injury, *biotrauma*. Biotrauma recognizes that mechanical ventilation is intrinsically pro-inflammatory and measures must be taken to minimize it.

High oxygen concentrations are known to result in lung injury. At the start of mechanical ventilation, the oxygen concentration of inspired air should be at 100% ($FiO_2 = 1.0$), and then weaned to 40–60% ($FiO_2 = 0.4–0.6$) as soon as possible to avoid oxygen toxicity. Oxygen toxicity rarely occurs at FiO_2 below 0.6.

Tidal volumes are initiated at $\sim$ 6–8 cc/kg to keep PIP $\leq$35 cm H_2O to minimize barotrauma. Normal minute ventilation (tidal volume x respiratory rate) should be approximately 100–150 cc/kg.

Monitoring

For all mechanically ventilated patients, capnometry (to measure end-tidal CO_2) is becoming a common monitoring tool. The end-tidal CO_2 allows the clinician to assess the integrity of the mechanical ventilation circuit. Levels can be trended. A positive slope suggests lower airway disease and a high baseline suggests auto-PEEP and air trapping that must be addressed. All patients require pulse oximetry and cardiac monitoring. Daily chest X-rays should be considered.

Appendix C

Wound Healing and Care

Biology of Wound Healing
- First intention healing occurs when the surrounding tissue of a wound is cleanly incised, reapproximated and repaired without infection; closure of a wound healed by first intention is *Primary Wound Closure*
- Second intention healing is the reparative process that occurs in an open wound with the formation of granulation tissue and eventual coverage by epithelial cells
- Third intention healing occurs when a wound is allowed to remain open for 3–5 days, and then is surgically closed; this is often used for severely contaminated wounds or wounds with extensive tissue loss (e.g., skin grafting); closure of a wound healed by third intention is referred to as *Delayed Primary Closure*

Three Phases of Primary Wound Healing
- Substrate Phase (Lag Phase) which is characterized by a "controlled inflammation" of the wound with release of enzymes, fluid, and protein; accumulation of white blood cells and connective tissue cells; and increased proliferation and perfusion of capillaries
- Proliferative Phase is characterized by early migration of epithelial cells (epithelization) and development of granulation tissue (beefy-red tissue caused by tremendous proliferation of capillaries) into the wound
- Resorptive Phase starts about 5–9 days after the injury and is characterized by wound contraction, collagen synthesis, and increased tissue strength

Factors Contributing to Poor Wound Healing
- Poor nutritional state
- Anemia
- Hypoproteinemia
- Hypovitaminosis
- Presence of debilitating diseases (e.g., diabetes, cancer, renal disease, chronic pulmonary disease)
- Steroid use
- Surgical local factors (e.g., poor tissue handling, poor hemostasis, infection, wound tension, foreign bodies, drains)

Definitions of Terms in Wound Healing and Care
- Primary wound closure – surgical closure and repair of a wound done soon after injury; wound heals by first intention (see "Biology of Wound Healing" above)
- Delayed primary closure – closure of a wound that has remained opened for several days and allowed to heal by secondary intention (see "Biology of Wound Healing" above)
- Debridement – physical removal of debris, infected tissue, necrotic tissue, and foreign material from a wound; can be done surgically (excision) or mechanically (irrigation or dressing changes)
- Wet-to-dry dressings – slightly moistened gauze dressing applied to a wound to facilitate mechanical debridement of dry, adherent wound debris; gauze dressing is allowed to dry out after several hours and removed to mechanically debride the gauze-adherent debris off of the wound surface (see "Wound and Surgical Dressings" below)
- Dehiscence – breakdown of wound; usually refers to fascial dehiscence of abdominal or thoracic wounds implying that the fascial or muscular closure has disrupted and broken down
- Evisceration – exposure and/or protrusion of an abdominal or thoracic organ through a wound; usually associated with a postoperative fascial dehiscence leading to skin and wound disruption with evisceration of underlying organ(s)

Appendix C

Wound and Surgical Dressings

- A fresh, clean surgical wound usually becomes epithelized within hours of closure; a dry, sterile, gauze dressing is commonly used to cover the wound, but is probably not necessary after 4–6 hours of closure
- Wounds with raw surface areas (e.g., abrasions) are covered with a non-adherent dressing (e.g., telfa or impregnated gauze dressings)
- Infected wounds or chronically draining wounds are often improved with frequent dressing changes
- Moist, draining wounds are best dressed with dry, absorbent gauze dressings, changed frequently
- Dry, open wounds with adherent debris and eschar formation may require moist dressings to facilitate wound care *(wet-to-dry dressings)* and allowed to dry over several hours; with each dressing change, this will mechanically debride the wound
- "If it's dry, wet it; if it's wet, dry it!"
- Gas-permeable, water-Impermeable plastic dressings are readily commercially available for fresh, clean surgical wounds

Appendix D

Surgical Drains and Tubes

Indications for the Use of Surgical Drains
- Provides a means for drainage of a contained abscess
- Decreases the risk of fluid collection or abscess after a surgical procedure
- Insecure closure of an intestinal perforation (e.g., perforation of an ulcer in a chronically scarred duodenum) where leak or fistula formation is possible
- In situations where a necrotic organ (e.g., pancreas) cannot be safely removed

Caveats
- It is impossible to drain the peritoneal cavity (e.g., in cases of diffuse peritonitis)
- Drains are a "two-way street"; they are a pathway for bacteria to migrate back into the surgical field or cavity
- The longer a drain is left in place, the greater the risk of secondary infection and/or erosion into adjacent organs or vessels
- Single lumen tubes (e.g., red rubber catheters) that require attachment to a suction device will suck adjacent bowel wall or the wall of abscess cavity against the end of the catheter; therefore, these tubes should be placed to intermittent suction
- Dual lumen tubes (sump) have an inner cannula or passage which allow circulation of air and fluids while attached to suction; may be placed on continuous suction
- Drains may lead to a false sense of security; bleeding or intestinal leak may occur with a drain in place but not come out of the drain, leading to delayed diagnosis and treatment

Definitions
- Open drain – a tube or drain that lies within a cavity or space and empties through an exit site onto the skin or a dressing; mostly soft, single lumen drains (e.g., Penrose drain) that passively drain fluid or pus; not good for removing debris or necrotic tissue; may only drain overflow fluid; especially prone to retrograde infection secondary to bacteria migrating along the drain
- Closed suction drains (e.g., Jackson-Pratt^R drain, Blake^R drains): Usually a soft, pliable, plastic drain that is connected to a closed suction system (usually a compressible bulb) that actively provides continuous negative pressure and serves as a reservoir to collect drainage; although retrograde infection can occur with a closed suction drain, the incidence is considerably less than with open drains
- Sump drains are firmer, larger drains that have an inner cannula, or passageway, that allows air or fluid to continuously circulate while attached to suction; these drains allow for better removal of necrotic tissue and debris; however, there is an increased risk of erosion into adjacent organs or vessels
- Percutaneously placed drainage catheters are now commonly placed by radiologists into fluid collections or abscess cavities via ultrasound or CT guidance

Special Tubes in Surgery
- Chest tube (tube thoracostomy) is a rigid drainage tube that is placed into the pleural space for decompression or evacuation of air and/or blood; commonly used to treat pneumothorax, hemothorax, and following thoracic surgery (e.g., pulmonary resection); chest tubes are connected to an underwater seal system to allow for the egress of fluid, air, or blood and to prevent the entry of air back into the pleural space
- Gastrostomy tube is a single or multi lumen tube placed into the stomach and exiting through the abdominal wall; used for gastric feeding or gastric decompression
    - Stamm gastrostomy: Tube is sewn into stomach wall and brought out through a stab wound in abdominal wall
    - Janeway gastrostomy: A small portion of the stomach wall is surgically partitioned to create a gastric tube; this portion of gastric tube is directly sutured to the skin, creating a permanent gastric-cutaneous fistula

—Percutaneous endoscopic gastrostomy (PEG): Gastrostomy tube is placed through the abdominal wall into the stomach via a percutaneous technique assisted with a gastroscope
- Jejunostomy tube is a surgically inserted tube into the proximal jejunum for feeding purposes; useful if unable to feed into stomach or duodenum (e.g., severe reflux, stomach or duodenal malignancy)
- T tube is a T-shaped silastic or latex tube designed for insertion into the common bile or common hepatic ducts; the limbs of the T are inserted above and below the dochotomy and bile drains out the long stem through an incision out of the abdominal wall
- Nasogastric tube is a semi-rigid sump tube used to decompress (and occasionally feed) the stomach; sump nasogastric tubes are attached to continuous suction for aspiration and drainage of gastric contents
- Other miscellaneous tubes sometimes encountered in surgery include cholecystostomy (gallbladder) tubes, cystostomy (bladder) tubes, cecostomy (cecum) tubes, and nephrostomy (renal pelvis) tubes

Index

Index

Index

Index

Index

Index

Index

Index

Index

Index

Index

Index

Index

Spinal cord compression, 155
Spinal cord injury, as differential diagnosis, 85, 86
Spinal stenosis, 157
Spindle cell nevi, 74
Spine tumor, as differential diagnosis, 157
Spleen injury, 88
Splenic artery, 46
Splenic vein thrombosis, as differential diagnosis, 31
Spondylosis, 156
Spontaneous intracerebral hematoma, as differential diagnosis, 150
Spontaneous perforation of bile duct, as differential diagnosis, 174
Spontaneous pneumothorax, 129
Squamous cell carcinoma, 71
  in bladder cancer, 116
  as differential diagnosis, 72, 74, 104, 105, 106
  in esophageal cancer, 8
  in lung cancer, 132
  in upper respiratory tumors, 134
Stab wounds, 89
Staghorn calculi, 123
Stamm gastrostomy, 186
Stanford classification of aortic dissection, 55
Staphylococcus
  infections associated with burns, 75
  infections in hidradenitis suppurativa, 69
  in liver abscesses, 32
  in prostatitis, 114
  See also Methicillin-resistant *Staphylococcus aureus* (MRSA)
Staphylococcus aureus
  in acute sinusitis, 102
  in lung abscesses, 130
  in osteomyelitis, 164
  in pilonidal disease, 70
  in septic arthritis, 165
Staphylococcus epidermidis
  in empyema, 128
  in osteomyelitis, 164
Stomach
  anatomy and function of, 2
  herniation of, 9
Strangulated inguinal hernia, as differential diagnosis, 120
Strangulation, 78
Streptococcal pneumoniae, in lung abscesses, 130
Streptococcus
  infections associated with burns, 75
  in liver abscesses, 32
  See also Group A *Streptococcus*
  See also Group B *Streptococcus*
Streptococcus pneumoniae
  in acute sinusitis, 102
  in septic arthritis, 165

Streptococcus pyogenes, in septic arthritis, 165
Streptococcus viridans, in empyema, 128
Stress fracture, as differential diagnosis, 161, 166
Stress incontinence, 122
Strictures
  as differential diagnosis, 6
  See also specific body system
Stroke, 57
  as differential diagnosis, 149
Struma ovarii, as differential diagnosis, 99
Struvite stones, 123
Subarachnoid hemorrhage (SAH), 148
  as differential diagnosis, 149
Subcutaneous fat, 68
Subdural hematoma, 85, 150
  as differential diagnosis, 149
Subluxation, 161
Subphrenic abscess, as differential diagnosis, 32
Substrate phase of wound healing, 184
Sump drains, 186
Superficial basal cell carcinoma, 72
Superficial femoral artery, 52
Superior laryngeal nerve paralysis, 108
Superior mesenteric artery, 2
Superior vena cava (SVC) obstruction, as differential diagnosis, 127
Surgical drains and tubes, 186–187
Surgical dressings, 185
Surgical thyroid disease, 99
Synchronized intermittent mandatory ventilation (SIMV), 182
Syncope, as differential diagnosis, 50, 140
Synovial cyst, as differential diagnosis, 157
Syphilis, as differential diagnosis, 70
Syphilitic chancre, as differential diagnosis, 24

T tube, 41, 187
Takayasu's arteritis, as differential diagnosis, 57
Telangiectasia, 68
  as cause of GI bleeding, 4
Tendon injury, as differential diagnosis, 161
Tension pneumothorax, 87, 129
Teratoma, 133
Testes, 110
Testicular agenesis, as differential diagnosis, 178
Testicular injury, 90
Testicular torsion, 120
  as differential diagnosis, 80, 117, 119
Testicular torsion, intrauterine, as differential diagnosis, 178
Testicular trauma, as differential diagnosis, 119
Testicular tumors, 117
  as differential diagnosis, 117, 118, 119, 120
Thermal burns, 75

Index

Index